The Truth About Senility—and How to Avoid It

Other books by Lawrence Galton

The Complete Medical, Health & Fitness Guide for Men

The Complete Medical Guide (with Benjamin F. Miller, M.D.)

Heart Attack: A Question & Answer Book (with Oscar Roth, M.D.)

Medical Advances

The Patient's Guide to Surgery

The Complete Book of Symptoms and What They Mean

Save Your Stomach

The Truth About Fiber in Your Food

Hypothyroidism: The Unsuspected Illness (with Broda O. Barnes, M.D.)

The Silent Disease: Hypertension

Freedom from Backaches (with Lawrence W. Friedmann, M.D.)

Adult Physical Fitness, The President's Council on Physical Fitness

The Truth About *SENILITY – and* How to Avoid It

Lawrence Galton

THOMAS Y. CROWELL, PUBLISHERS

Established 1834

New York

Designer: Stephanie Winkler

Library of Congress Cataloging in Publication Data

Galton, Lawrence.
   The truth about senility—and how to avoid it.
   1. Senile psychosis. 2. Geriatric
psychiatry. 3. Aged—Psychology. I. Title.
RC524.G34   1979   618.9′76′89   79–7086
ISBN 0–690–01833–9

   80 81 82 83 10 9 8 7 6 5 4 3 2

Contents

Preface

What can you expect as you grow older—or watch someone else do so?

What really is inevitable—and what not—with aging?

Must there be that most devastating and frightening disease of aging—senility—which destroys a person's memory, reasoning, personality?

Compelling as these questions have always been—now even more so as more people live to older ages—they have, until very recently, been left largely unanswered—unanswered, that is, in any reliable sense. There has been no shortage of myths.

Finally, we are beginning to get valid—and rewarding—answers.

The aim of this book is to provide a clear picture of what modern research has been uncovering about what does and does not happen with aging, what is inevitable and what is not, and how relatively rare is true senile dementia with which senility is commonly equated.

It will show you the pseudosenilities—in which impairments of mental functioning and disturbances of behavior are severe enough to seem like true dementia yet are really due to physical influences in the body that may be far removed from the brain itself, and occasionally to psychological factors.

And, in considering these influences, you will find that many can be prevented from developing and operating, others when already present can be overcome before they have a chance to impair. Not least of all, you will also find that correction of such causes, once recognized, may well rescue someone now classified as "hopelessly" senile.

The Truth About Senility—and How to Avoid It

1

Senility: Fear, Fancy, Fact

To no small extent, a once almost universal fear—of early death—today has been replaced by another: of senility and confused, doddering, useless, suffering, vegetative old age.

Forget much if not all you may have thought you knew about senility.

There is now a large, even if not yet generally appreciated, body of evidence, thanks to recent research, that

1. Senility is *not* a natural accompaniment of old age, something to be expected, an inevitable part of the aging process;

2. Although real senility does exist, it is far less common than supposed; and when it does exist, it is not invariably beyond all help; and

3. Much of what is called senility is not senility at all but rather pseudosenility, which can be avoided and when present can often be erased.

I know that this goes against much or even all of what we have long heard and come to believe, of what has to some extent been transmitted to us as a kind of cultural heritage.

The Historic Picture

"Youth," wrote the Greek poet Euripides, who lived more than 400 years before Christ, "is always dear to me; old age is a load that lies more heavily on the head than the rocks of Elna."

1

Sophocles, too, complained: "All evils are ingrained in long old age; lost wits, unprofiting action, empty thoughts." And this, even as he himself lived to ninety and continued busy and creatively productive to the end.

A pessimistic view of old age is represented by an old Yiddish gibe based on the Hebrew word for old age, *zokon,* which, as Dr. Harry A. Savitz of Beth Israel Hospital, Boston, has pointed out, "is ironically abbreviated to read Ziphzen, which means sighing, Krechzen, which means groaning, Nissen, which means sneezing, and Husten, which means coughing."

But beyond the cultural heritage of the past, we have a contemporary mythology.

The Modern Stereotype

Dr. Robert N. Butler is the director of the new National Institute on Aging, which is part of the U.S. Government's National Institutes of Health. Before that, Butler was research psychiatrist and gerontologist for the Washington School of Psychiatry.

Twenty years ago, Butler drew up a sketch that stereotyped old age. Reviewing it recently, he found that it hasn't changed much.

This is the stereotype in Butler's words:

"An older person thinks and moves slowly. He does not think as he used to, nor as creatively. He is bound to himself and to his past and can no longer change or grow. He can neither learn well nor swiftly, and even if he could, he would not wish to. Tied to his personal traditions and growing conservatism, he dislikes innovations and is not disposed to new ideas. Not only can he not move forward, he often moves backwards.

"He enters a second childhood, caught often in increasing egocentricity and demanding more from his environment than he is willing to give to it. Sometimes he becomes more like himself, a caricature of a lifelong personality. He becomes irritable and cantankerous, yet shallow and enfeebled. He lives in his past. He is behind the times. He is aimless and wandering of mind, reminiscing and garrulous. Indeed, he is a study in decline. He is the picture of mental and physical failure.

"He is often stricken by diseases which in turn restrict his movement, his enjoyment of food, the pleasures of well-being. His sexual interest and activity decline. His body shrinks; so, too, does the flow of blood to his brain. His mind does not utilize oxygen and sugar at the same rate as formerly. Feeble, uninteresting, he awaits his death, a burden to society, to his family, and to himself."

The Alarming Statistics

To go with the stereotype, you may have seen what appear to be distressing current statistics, figures to make you wonder what if any chance you have of living any reasonably happy kind of later years.

For example:

- That illness becomes an ever-increasing problem for the elderly, with those over sixty-five twice as likely as younger people to suffer from one or more chronic conditions;
- That 42 percent of the elderly have some limitation on activity because of chronic conditions;
- That people over sixty-five spend more than three times as much time in hospital as do younger people;
- That the elderly use three times as many prescription drugs as well as an unaccountable number of nonprescription preparations.

Quite likely, too, you have heard about vast numbers of older people confined to institutions or withering away in nursing homes, their brains diseased, suffering from confusion, memory impairment, emotional lability, paranoid delusions, loss of orientation, illusions and hallucinations, some of them completely apathetic and withdrawn, others agitated, assaultive and irascible, many of them wandering off, accidentally injuring themselves, incontinent.

Bleak picture? But not when viewed in perspective and with some correction.

A Better Perspective . . .
and an Emerging New Picture

Certainly, physical changes occur with aging. Some are obvious; some not necessarily apparent. There are many changes.

But the changes do not in themselves spell disease.

The elderly do, indeed, have more illnesses than young people, but those illnesses, we now know, are not the result of aging. When they come, it is because they often had their inception in younger years; very often, they have been neglected or mistreated; and very often they still remain amenable to either cure or otherwise helpful treatment.

Do all elderly people become senile?

Obviously not. Undoubtedly, you know of many examples of achievement in later years: Benjamin Franklin writing his autobiography when over eighty; Stradivarius still making his violins up to the age of ninety-three; Grandma Moses beginning to paint at seventy-nine; Michelangelo completing his painting on the ceiling of the Sistine Chapel when he was over eighty; Verdi producing *Falstaff* at eighty; Agatha Christie writing novels in her eighties; David Ben-Gurion active through his mid-eighties; and Mao Tse-tung, DeValera, Mahatma Gandhi, Marshal Tito, Pablo Casals, Rubinstein, Stokowski, and many more too numerous to count who reflect, if anything, the triumph of aging.

But do *most* elderly people become senile?

No. However, because many have various symptoms less common in younger people, they are frequently regarded as senile by their acquaintances, their families, and even their physicians.

Actually, only 4 to 5 percent of the older population are so impaired as to be institutionalized. And many of these do not really need to be.

Unhappily, too often physicians have tended to interpret many reversible and treatable disorders as irreversible dementia, thus denying the elderly the right to treatment.

"Go to any general hospital or nursing home," says Dr. Edward Dreyfus, interim director of the new research-oriented Davis Institute for the Care and Study of the Aging in Denver, "and see catch-all diagnoses of 'senility' in the patients' charts. Most so labeled actually have disease that is treatable. This wastebasket term is a condemnation to a neglected life of despair and for no reason."

Vignettes

- In a case now become something of a classic, a sixty-six-year-old man, a once-prominent judge, is admitted to a New York hospital, apparently hopelessly senile, and so considered for two years during which he has become increasingly confused, disoriented, with large memory deficits, and growing paranoid suspiciousness. Surgery to overcome hydrocephalus ("water on the brain")—and more on this later—makes him alert, cheerful, oriented, able to function normally within forty-eight hours.
- They are three elderly women, all with the trappings of senility—but not hopeless. They have three different underlying problems: one, a gland disorder; the second, a disorder of the same gland but in the opposite direction; the third, a grossly elevated blood-fat condition for the first time linked to bizarre behavioral changes. All respond to treatment.
- She is seventy-two, confused, apathetic, withdrawn, taking no interest in anything, sitting for hours just staring into

space, often giving no indication that she hears when spoken to. Hopelessly senile? No. Her problem: mental depression. It yields to treatment.

These are just a few of the many examples you will be reading about later in this book.

They indicate more than that seeming senility can—and very often does—result from treatable disease. They also underscore the opportunities for prevention.

Many years ago, in a different context, de Tocqueville observed, "The evil which was suffered patiently as inevitable seems unendurable as soon as the idea of escaping from it crosses men's minds."

So it should be with any notion that we must inevitably with aging lapse into a useless vegetative state.

2

The Changes That Do—and Do Not—Occur with Aging

Many changes do, of course, take place with the passing of years. Some are quite obvious. Wrinkles appear on the skin and so may brown (so-called liver) spots. The hair becomes grayer and perhaps thinner.

Vision changes are among the first that make people aware of aging. Glasses for reading and close work are very commonly needed after age forty because of presbyopia, which results from loss of the ability of the lens to accommodate for near and distant vision.

In advanced years, vision also may be affected by a slowing of adaptation to darkness and a need for increased illumination. Older people often do not see objects clearly in light at as low a level as do younger people and may require brighter light for some tasks.

Cataracts—opaque spots that form on the lens of the eye and impair vision—are not unique to the elderly; they occur in some young people because of injuries, exposure to heat or radiation, or inherited factors, but in most cases they are called senile cataracts and appear to be part of the aging process for some people. They are, of course, correctable by surgery at any age.

Interestingly, Dr. Mortimer Shapiro of Mount Sinai School of Medicine, New York City, has suggested that since vision is responsible for over half of a person's sensory input, diminishing vision with age may help to explain why older people tend to retain their earlier obtained and more youthful view of things.

Other Perceptual Changes

With aging, hearing acuity may diminish to some degree. Hearing loss is not always as readily apparent to the individual as vision impairment, although it often is to those around him. One reason for this, it has been suggested, is that all of us with normal hearing guess some sounds without necessarily realizing that we are guessing. Older people with hearing impairment may do much more guessing, and they may often make erroneous guesses.

Typically, this hearing alteration in later years—called presbycusis—is characterized by reduced ability to distinguish high frequency sounds. This may be an aging process. But all hearing impairment in older people may not be age-related. Some studies have indicated that hearing loss does not occur in primitive societies. Dr. Samuel Rosen, a New York hearing specialist, has studied a Sudanese tribe, the Mabaan, and found that their hearing is as keen at age seventy as it is in most Americans at seventeen. There are indications that exposure to high noise levels is detrimental to Americans.

In some older people, hearing loss is caused by a problem that develops in some younger people: otosclerosis, a hardening of a middle ear bone, the stapes, which conducts sound vibrations. With hardening, the bone becomes rigid and unable to transmit vibratory sound waves. Stapedectomy—a surgical procedure in which the stapes is removed and replaced with a prosthesis—is highly successful in many older as well as younger people.

Other senses may be impaired to some degree. Taste buds on the tongue, which are constantly replaced throughout life, may in some older people be replaced less rapidly, leading to diminished taste sense. The first buds to be affected are those on the front of the tongue that detect sweet and salty, leaving those that detect bitter and sour tastes. This appears to be why some older people complain that all foods taste bitter or sour.

Smell sensitivity, too, may be reduced. In one study of 256 "normal" elderly subjects, with a mean age of 70.8 years, only 32 percent were found to have olfactory ability comparable to that of young adults. In one-fourth, olfaction was slightly diminished; in 42 percent it was greatly diminished. Over 50 percent of people sixty-five years of age or older reportedly cannot smell domestic gas (in one study, over 75 percent of 892 deaths due to domestic gas poisoning were of people over sixty years of age).

Are diminished taste and smell the result of aging per se? As yet, there is no definitive answer. Some investigators believe yes; others hold that the losses result from smoking and disease. And it should be noted that in some cases investigators have found taste and smell disturbances in people with thyroid gland disorder (hypothyroidism) which have responded to thyroid treatment, and in other instances other investigators have found many people whose gustatory senses responded remarkably to treatment with zinc sulfate to make up for zinc deficiency.

Sensory changes may have psychological repercussions. If an older person loses more and more acuity, particularly of sight or hearing, and is unaware of the loss or refuses to admit it or do anything about it, he or she, no longer experiencing old satisfactions, may tend to withdraw from old activities.

Other Changes

Many older people, particularly women, shrink somewhat in height as the result of loss of collagen, a fibrous protein, between the vertebrae of the spine. Such shrinkage in some cases may begin as early as age twenty or thirty.

With aging there is likely to be a gradual decline in muscular strength. Such strength may reach its peak by or before age thirty; and baseball and football players, boxers, and track athletes seldom perform as well after thirty as before.

Actually, the cells that make up the voluntary muscles may diminish in number with age, so that by the age of eighty only about half may be left. As muscle cells disappear, they are replaced by fat and fibrous connective tissue.

Exercise, of course, may help counter this; but the effects of exercise here have not as yet been studied in detail.

Both men and women lose bone after age forty. But women lose far more than men. The rate of loss per decade is about 3 percent in men and 8 percent in women.

Lung function declines with age. For example, the maximal breathing capacity—the amount of air moved through the lungs in fifteen seconds—is reduced by 40 percent between the ages of twenty and eighty years. Obesity and weakening of muscles that lift the rib cage for breathing may contribute to reduced lung function. And there is a question of how much exposure to lung disease and pollution, cigarette smoke, and other environmental influences may contribute to aging of the lungs.

Some investigators have found that a decrease in heart output begins at about age twenty, and with advancing age there may be other changes. But the aged heart is not necessarily a diseased organ. However, as in the young, such conditions as high blood pressure and hardening of the coronary arteries feeding the heart may lead to a state of disease.

High levels of cholesterol in the blood, which are considered risk factors for coronary artery disease and heart attacks, seem to peak at about age fifty-five. In a study at the Gerontology Research Center of the National Institute of Aging in Baltimore, subjects up to age fifty-five, on the average, had an increasing amount of cholesterol in the blood, while those surviving beyond fifty-five showed a decrease.

Much yet remains to be learned about the effects of aging on the gastrointestinal system. Some older people complain of dryness of the mouth, which may result from a decreased flow of saliva. It is known that the stomach tends to secrete less hydro-chloric acid with aging. Some studies have shown that absorption of calcium—a mineral needed for healthy bones in particular—may begin to fall off starting at age fifty-five to sixty in women and sixty-five to seventy in men. The extent to which vitamin D deficiency might be involved in this has not yet been evaluated. There is also some evidence indicating that with aging there may be a decrease in the ability to digest protein.

Only a few people beyond the age of seventy are entirely free of kidney changes. Blood flow through the kidneys may be reduced.

There are conflicting reports about how common prostate enlargement may be among older men. Some studies indicate that about 30 percent of the male population will have some enlargement at age sixty or beyond; others indicate some degree of enlargement in as many as 76 percent of those over age fifty-five.

Metabolism means the sum of all the chemical reactions that take place in the body. It is estimated that the basic metabolic rate declines about 16 percent from age thirty to age seventy, while the caloric requirements—because of decreased exercise as well as metabolism—may drop about one-third.

Drugs are handled differently in older people than in younger. This is due to the decline in metabolism, which includes such processes as absorption, distribution, destruction, and excretion of drugs. And as muscle cells are replaced by fat and fibrous connective tissue, the latter provide increased storage capacity for drugs so that more may be retained.*

Sleep patterns change with age. Older people generally take

---

* A study sponsored by the National Institute on Aging has shown that older men generally handle alcohol as well as younger men physiologically, but there are differences in metabolism. The same amount of alcohol, for example, produced a higher peak blood alcohol level in older men. Physiologically, older men appeared less intoxicated than their younger counterparts, but testing showed that their memory and decision-making ability were impaired more than in younger subjects. Since alcohol has greater psychological effects on the old and they perceive those effects to a lesser degree, the drug is potentially more risky for older men than for younger ones.

longer to fall asleep, their sleep is lighter, and they have more frequent awakenings. It can be important that older people recognize that these changes are normal and no cause for concern.

Brain Changes

The discovery some years ago that beginning shortly after the age of twenty we apparently lose, every day, 50,000 neurons (nerve cells) of the brain and nervous system seemed disconcerting.

But that loss, if it really occurs, need hardly be disturbing. It would certainly appear that the number of cells lost and the number remaining are not nearly as important as the number actually used.

Observes Dr. George G. Haydu of the Creedmoor Institute for Psychobiologic Studies, Queens Village, New York: "Function is the criterion. It would be quite contrary to carefully documented studies to think that psychological functions and activities are on the downgrade after the age of twenty. Indeed, our abilities in problem solving, concept formation, availability of knowledge, and the sensing and use of appropriate means and time, grow continually after the age of twenty while undoubtedly thousands of neurons die every day."

And Haydu goes on to point out that it seems we have a huge reserve of neurons available for use, and this is hardly an exception in biology. Lung capacity, kidney capacity, liver function capabilities, and many others are greatly in excess of actual need.

Actually, whether the brain's higher centers lose large numbers of brain cells has been brought into question very recently by Dr. Marian C. Diamond, professor of anatomy at the University of California, Berkeley.

Early in 1978, writing in *American Scientist,* Dr. Diamond reported that studies by many scientists now indicate that "there is good evidence that drastic structural changes do not occur in the mammalian brain with aging," provided the animal lives in a stimulating environment.

In her report, Dr. Diamond cited her own recent study in which nerve cells in the cerebral cortices of male rats, living three per cage, were counted in young, adult, and old rats. No significant loss of cells could be found in adult and old rats.

In previous aging studies in which such a loss was indicated, Dr. Diamond noted, investigators did not always consider the importance of environmental living conditions of the aging animals, or of people when they were the subjects of study.

Diamond argues that if we dare "extrapolate results found in rats to human beings," then, "as long as the brain is exposed to a stimulating environment," structural changes such as brain cell loss are probably less significant than role experiences, psychosocial relationships, and other environmental factors in determining well-being and personality. "In the absence of disease, impoverished environment, or poor nutrition," Dr. Diamond concludes, "the nervous system apparently does have the potential to oppose marked deterioration with aging."

The Mental Decline Myth

More and more recent studies have upset, scientifically, an old—and to some extent still popularly prevalent—notion of a peaking of human intellectual capacity early in life followed by gradual diminution until, so the myth would have it, it has fallen very low by the sixties.

For example, some years ago the National Institute of Mental Health followed a group of men as they moved from an average age of seventy-one to eighty-one years. The study found a "remarkably high quality of mental functioning" despite advanced age. Retests at the end of the ten years showed performances remaining close to what they had been to begin with.

In the words of the study report, published in 1971, "Declines, of course, are evident, but what stands out are the residual capabilities. . . . This is a matter which has received relatively limited attention in gerontological research reports. Yet, from both a practical and theoretical standpoint in understanding and dealing with advanced aging, it is crucial to consider the resources which the individual possesses, along with his potential for both reinforcing and extending them. . . . The aged may be getting less credit than they deserve for the extent of their intellectual, perceptual, and personality strengths and capabilities."

Older people may not do well where rapid response is called for, but when the pace of a learning task is slowed, the elderly improve markedly in performance. On some intellectual tasks, in fact, there may even be an increase in capability with age. Stored information, of course, is continually mounting with the years. If, say, as a college graduate you may have known 20,000 words, it is likely that you may know twice that number by age sixty-five.

But if stored knowledge increases, searching for it and retrieving it tend to proceed more slowly. Quick response is an attribute of the young, and they clearly do better than the aged under time pressure. However, when given opportunity to make maximum use of their experience and knowledge on a self-paced basis, the elderly do very well—a reason why, for instance, writing is a skill that often flourishes late in life.

Nor is there any need for the elderly—and many undoubtedly would be helped if they realized this—to be embarrassed about a slowing which appears to be a normal part of aging and no indication of mental decline.

Perhaps Dr. James E. Birren, director of the University of Southern California's Ethel and Percy Andrus Gerontology Center, has put it as well as anyone:

"I don't feel particularly embarrassed if someone should tell me that I don't process as much information per unit of time as I used to. This is no ego blow to me.

"There is a concept I use to help me over any residual ego concern that may be involved in the fact that I am no longer as good an information processor. I explain the change using a conceptual approach. . . . If you have a secretary who puts letters in a file as they come in, you will have a complete chronological file, but one where it's difficult to have easy access to any one letter. So access time lengthens purely as a function of the amount stored. In our brains we take care of this filing problem by organizing information into a conceptual store. What were previously discrete bits of information now form a concept group. You reach through the concept to relevant experience.

"Let's take a practical example. We did interviewing at the University of Chicago of successful middle-aged men and women. One of the things they talked about is that they had come to deal with professional matters with less intensity in middle age. A high school principal said, "When I started out, each disciplinary problem in the school was a special problem for me. I intervened; I went all out for it. Now I withdraw a little more and let the teacher handle it until I can see what is going on." As another example, the firstborn child is a big crisis for the man and the woman. The first time the baby cries at home, the mother cries. There is much emotional involvement. This is not so with the second and third child. If only mothers could begin with their fourth child, then they could deal with the issues conceptually. With maturation comes a greater conceptual grasp so that we can size up the situation and then look to the relevant items in our store. This is what I call the race between the chunks and the bits. While younger people, say those between eighteen and twenty-two, can process more bits per second, and even though by age sixty, that number may be halved, the older person may process bigger chunks. The race may go to the tortoise because he is chunking, and not to the hare because he is just bitting along."

The idea that learning ability and even IQ must drop as a

natural consequence of old age has been challenged by many investigators recently.

At the respected Jackson Laboratory in Bar Harbor, Maine, Dr. Richard L. Sprott has been carrying out careful behavioral studies with animals. He has observed the same types of animals in maximum-learning environments through much of their life span: from five weeks, which is comparable to human childhood, to thirty months, which is equal to post-retirement age.

He has found that 90 percent of the animals in one group and 80 percent in another group learned as well in very old age as they did when they were very much younger.

Learning ability and IQ, instead of decreasing with age, remain steady and perhaps even increase, Sprott is convinced, depending on an individual's profession, interests, and health.

Says Dr. George G. Haydu in a report called "Aging and Experience Forms" published in the *New York State Journal of Medicine:* "We must realize that intelligence as measured by the Wechsler scale and similar instruments cannot be equated with the power and function of what we call the intellect. The latter is the capacity to see and manage, apply, combine, and recombine what the individual finds meaningful and significant in his world, which of course is his cultural world. This capacity does not suffer decline, except in terminal senescence. A reflection of this is the observation that even in the Wechsler scale, vocabulary and comprehension components stay high. One's comprehension, judgment, and understanding grow steadily well after the age of twenty."

Dr. E. David Sherman adds something more. Dr. Sherman, who is director of research at Montreal's Rehabilitation Institute, chairman of the Quebec Medical Association's Committee on Aging, and lecturer in geriatrics at the University of Montreal, reports: "General intelligence, once having reached its peak, can be maintained at this level even into old age, *especially if the person continues to be active and shows no deterioration* associated with extensive physical and neurological changes." (The italics are Dr. Sherman's.)

"Since education," he goes on, "fosters maintenance of intellectual ability, continued learning throughout life presumably would have a similar effect. A high level of intelligence, a good education, and continuous practice in exercising the capacity to learn, appear to delay the onset of any loss of ability to learn. Memory for past events appears to be less impaired than retention and recall of recent experiences. Failure of immediate recall, perhaps associated with inability to register what is new, characterizes memory impairment in old age. Aged people who are in good health, however, show much less deficit in short-term memory than do those who are in poor health."

And Sherman also notes, "The effects of aging are not uniform. As certain physical attributes decline with age, others become stronger. Memory may decline, but judgment concerning the significance of the facts improves with age. Visual acuity diminishes, but the ability to comprehend what is seen improves with experience. Experience is dependent upon time, and therefore inevitably grows with age."

Creativity and Productivity

There are many examples to indicate that old age is not inevitably a barrier for creative people. At eighty, Tennyson wrote "Crossing the Bar." Michelangelo was eighty-nine when he painted some of his greatest masterpieces. Verdi was eight-five when he composed *Te Deum.* Viscount Bryce, who was over eighty when he published his two-volume *Modern Democracies,* upon the occasion of his addressing the Harvard student body, was introduced with the remark that "whenever Mr. Bryce might happen to die, he would die young."

Sir Winston Churchill even managed to triumph over breaking

all the rules of maintaining health—smoking cigars almost continuously, drinking champagne and brandy like water, keeping irregular hours, working under extreme tension—and yet living to ninety-one. Had he retired when he was sixty-five, which was in 1939, the Battle of Britain would have had to be fought without him.

In 1953, Churchill was rumored to have had a stroke, although the official word was that he had retired for a month's rest. Two years later, in the House of Commons, he admitted during a debate that he had had a stroke which had left him paralyzed and unable to speak; but he had overcome his disabilities and now, he warned his opponent, he would walk, talk, and fight as he always had.

Some years ago, Jack W. Taylor, director of executive development at Planning Dynamics, Inc., Pittsburgh, was able to refute a common reactionary view in industry that the human brain tends to stultify at some point after age thirty-five, and if a business is to achieve creative impetus it has to acquire "new" young minds.

Beyond pointing to scientific studies negating this hypothesis, Taylor instituted creativity-development programs in a number of major U.S. business organizations. In each program there were pretests of the creative ability of the participants, followed by training in the principles and techniques of creative thinking, and then testing to measure results of the training. Afterward, there was continuing follow-up to evaluate participants' subsequent creative contributions.

The greatest positive response as shown in performance in the post-training tests was made by older men, with average improvement of 146 percent for those older than forty as against 62 percent for those under thirty. And, most important, in the practical application phase extending over a period of many years, 80 percent of all the most worthwhile and workable new ideas came from those over forty.

What the programs suggest is that when it comes to creative

accomplishments and productivity, older people have the best of it for many reasons. At later ages, there is less waste and greater conservation and use of vital energy; activity is much more direct, controlled, and therefore efficient; older people are inured to work; they have the experience to avoid pitfalls and fads that often trap the young; they have the willpower and persistence needed for creative achievement; they bring greater continuity of attention, interest, and motivation to their work.

"Contrast all this," observes Taylor, "with the all-too-observable tendency of so many youngsters toward short attention spans . . . preoccupation with status, personal advancement, politicosocial relations, etc., rather than self-fulfillment . . . proclivity to 'reinventing the wheel,' not knowing what has already been tried . . . desire . . . to 'revolutionize the world without having to bother with the necessity of first building a working model' . . . and the like. And the contrast becomes sharp indeed!"

The Variability of Change

About one thing, all investigators of aging are in agreement: there is tremendous variation in the way people age, great individual differences in rates of aging.

Within the same individual, different organ systems age at different rates. A seventy-year-old may have a heart output no better than that for an eighty-year-old, while another may have an output to match that of a forty-year-old. But the seventy-year-old with the forty-year-old heart may have kidney function like that of an eighty-year-old.

There is at least as much difference between individual older people as between individual younger people. In fact, there is evidence that as people grow old they become even more diverse, more heterogeneous, than their juniors.

As one investigator has pointed out, and the observation is certainly within our own experience: "Some people are old in middle age, others young in old age."

The Alterability of Change

Are all of the changes associated with aging beyond control, not subject to being held in check or at least slowed?

That may be true of some, but clearly it is not true of all.

For one thing, it's apparent that on the whole older people today are physiologically younger than those of say seventy-five or eighty years ago. "Many of our sixty-five-year-olds today," notes Professor Walter M. Beattie, Jr., of Syracuse University, "are more like their fifty-year-old counterparts at the turn of the century, due to improved nutrition, health care, and environmental sanitation. Whistler's mother, who epitomizes 'old age,' was forty-four years of age when she sat for that famous painting."

Much of the deterioration once blamed on aging now, increasingly, appears to be the result of disease instead.

One example is atherosclerosis, which was once considered a normal part of the aging process. But it is now apparent that this disease of the arteries has nothing to do with age per se. It's a disease that can be found in young people. It progresses with time, but time doesn't cause it.

Many of the other so-called attributes of aging are being found to come with age but not because of age.

And we are beginning to see demonstrations of the alterability of some of these attributes.

For example, more youthful muscle tone and strength can be regained by sixty- to ninety-year-olds with an exercise program of six to eight weeks' duration.

Another example: Some of the irritability, fatigue, sleeping problems, and even confusion in the elderly have been reversed by improvement in diet.

Still another: Loss of bone density—osteoporosis—which is a common problem in the aged, particularly among women, may be less—if at all—a matter of aging and more or entirely a result of faulty diet and hormone imbalance. And the loss of calcium from bone, which is what is involved, has been markedly reduced in recent studies simply by putting more calcium into the diet.

And another: In the Baltimore study by the National Institute on Aging, heavy cigarette smoking has been shown to be related to reduced lung function in older people; and when smoking is stopped, the lung function returns to near normal within eighteen to twenty-four months.

When it comes to senility, certainly that cannot be an inevitable consequence of aging, since it does not occur in all older people, nor even in anything approaching a majority.

Says Dr. Eward W. Busse, a specialist in aging research at Duke University: "With the passage of time there are numerous biological changes in the human body and brain . . . but it does not appear that the older person who is physically healthy and mentally active inevitably progresses to intellectual losses and mental incapacity."

When true senile dementia occurs, it is because of disease. And when pseudodementia occurs, it is because of disease, often physical, sometimes psychological, very commonly treatable and even preventable.

3

True Senility (Dementia)

When Oliver Wendell Holmes was 92 years old
he was visited by Franklin D. Roosevelt, who found
him reading Plato. "Why do you read Plato, Mr.
Justice?" asked FDR. "To improve my mind, Mr.
President," was Holmes' reply.

—Medical Tribune

It would be gratifying if old age were invariably a time for improving the mind. But it is not—invariably.

True dementia does exist. It is not nearly as common as supposed. Although it is considered irreversible, it is often confused
with reversible conditions. And there is good reason to hope
that in many cases even the irreversible is treatable to a worthwhile extent.

Dementia is certainly not the same thing as the minor memory
loss or increased forgetfulness that sometimes may come with
old age.

Dementia can be insidious in onset. In the earliest stages,
the symptoms may be only exaggerations of presickness personality. There may be immoderate emotional responses to ordinary
daily affairs previously handled without difficulty. Previous ability
to carry out intellectual activities and solve problems may diminish. Interests may shrink, and there may be apathy which sometimes may alternate with irritability.

Not long after such changes occur, other declines in mental
functioning may become apparent. Difficulty in receiving, retain-
ing, and recalling new information may increase. A simple newly

acquired fact or bit of information may not be recalled even after only a few minutes. After watching a television news program or reading a newspaper, a patient may be unable to answer a question about what he or she has seen or read.

There may then follow progressive disorganization of personality, with disorientation for time, situation, and possibly even place—to the point where the patient no longer may recognize family members, old familiar places, or even self.

In one instance, for example, a man suffering from dementia was shown a photograph of a voluptuous woman in a bikini. Asked what he saw, he could only reply, "I know it isn't a tractor. But could it be a house?"

Sometimes a patient may lose so much ability to retain information that he cannot recall where he is or recite a few simple words, such as house, boat, umbrella, a few minutes after they are presented.

Major Forms

It happened more than half a century ago. The woman at first showed signs of difficulty in thinking, remembering, and speaking. The difficulty increased. Subsequently, she became pathologically jealous of her husband, took to hiding objects around the house, suffered an impairment in gait and thereafter a rapid sharp decline in her mental and physical state. When she died four and a half years later, she was only fifty-one years old.

She suffered from what is now known to have been Alzheimer's disease, named after the German neurologist who first described it. Until recently, the disease was thought to be a special, rare form of presenile dementia, striking people in their forties and fifties.

Today, however, brain studies with the electron microscope and other advanced techniques have convinced virtually all inves-

tigators that Alzheimer's in younger people and a large proportion of dementia in older people are identical.

Dementia also may stem from arteriosclerosis of brain blood
vessels which interferes with circulation to brain tissues.

In one study of fifty successive demented elderly patients coming to autopsy, Alzheimer's disease was found to account for
half of the cases, to have contributed equally in 8 percent with
arteriosclerosis, and to have possibly played some role in another
10 percent. Brain changes due to arteriosclerosis accounted definitely for 12 percent of the cases, probably for an additional 6
percent, contributed equally with Alzheimer's in 8 percent, and
played some role in 10 percent.

Alzheimer's Disease

Autopsies on the brains of senile patients after death have
shown some apparently critical differences but also some surprising similarities with the normal brain.

Surprisingly, an aged brain and a senile brain weigh about
the same. Both have ventricles, or spaces, of about the same
size. And, unexpectedly, investigators have found that the number of neurons or nerve cells in many areas of the brain do
not differ markedly.

But there is an area of the brain, the hippocampus, which is
known to be involved in memory storage. And very recently,
one investigator, Dr. J. A. N. Corsellis of Runwell Hospital in
Wickford, Essex, England, has reported finding a greatly reduced
number of neurons in the hippocampus.

Very recently, too, another striking deficit—in blood flow to
the hippocampus area—has been shown as the result of a dramatic technique for measuring cerebral blood flow developed
in the laboratory of Dr. David H. Ingvar of the University Hospital of Lund, Sweden. Radioactively labeled xenon is injected
into an artery (the carotid) supplying the brain. The xenon is
measured with a computerized detection device, and the mea-

surements are converted into a color-coded "photograph" of the brain.

The color differences indicate variations in blood flow, and Dr. Ingvar and his associates have observed reductions in blood flow to the hippocampus and other areas of the cerebral cortex of the brain in Alzheimer patients, with indications that the reductions are proportional to the degree of dementia.

An intriguing feature of the Swedish technique is that it can be used to visualize thought processes. For example, when a person is asked to close his eyes or is presented with a problem to solve, color changes indicating changes in blood flow can be seen on the computerized picture.

The technique, Dr. Ingvar reports, "represents a new means of diagnosing cerebral defects in the living patient."

The brain of a patient with Alzheimer's disease has other distinguishing features. One is the presence of plaques interspersed among the neurons in the brain. Plaques consist of aggregates of altered nerve fibers and an abnormal protein called amyloid.

Another feature is the presence within neurons of neurofibrillary tangles, abnormally changed fibrils or minute fibers that have become thickened, twisted, and distorted.

Actually, plaques begin to appear in middle age. They gradually increase with age and are found in about 70 percent of all people over sixty-five. But the number of plaques is limited in most intellectually normal people. The tangles also occur with increasing frequency in a few areas of the brain with aging, but their number remains small in other areas in normal older people.

In Alzheimer's disease, the plaques and tangles tend to be especially common in the hippocampus area.

Causes

In the summer of 1977, a special three-day workshop conference on Alzheimer's disease was sponsored by the National Institute on Aging and other institutes of the federal National Institutes of Health. It brought together scientists from around the world and is expected to be a first major step toward concentrating increased attention on determining the causes and possible means for combating the disease.

Already there are clues to causes.

There is evidence, for example, that there may be some genetic basis. One study of affected patients and their relatives found a 60 percent risk among identical twins, a 40 percent risk among fraternal twins, a 6 percent risk among siblings, and a 3 percent risk for parents of victims. Another study found a 10 percent risk for parents and a 4 percent risk for siblings—very much in excess of the risk in the general population.

Recently, too, senility—along with Down's syndrome (mongolism) and leukemia—has been found to cluster in some families. And at the 1977 conference, Dr. F. C. Stam of Vrije University in Amsterdam reported finding three blood proteins, called haptoglobins, to be especially prevalent in senility patients. The proteins are controlled by genes all on a single chromosome (number 16). Stam also reported that people with the proteins are more at risk for leukemia.

Several investigators have found evidence of impaired message transmission in Alzheimer's disease. In the brain and central nervous system, messages travel from one neuron to the next, across gaps between the neurons, with the aid of chemicals called neurotransmitters.

For some of these neurons—called cholinergic neurons—the neurotransmitter is acetylcholine. In recent studies in Britain, Dr. Peter Davies of the Thomas Clouston Clinic in Edinburgh and Dr. Alan N. Davison of the National Hospital in London found in the brains of patients with Alzheimer's disease a significant depletion of an enzyme (cholineacetyltransferase) which is needed for cholinergic neurons to produce acetylcholine. And the depletion is particularly pronounced in the hippocampus.

A promising task for research, according to Dr. Robert Terry, chairman of pathology at New York's Albert Einstein College of Medicine, may be to learn how to induce the brain to produce the vital enzyme, perhaps with a drug.

In this same area, Dr. David Drachman of Northwestern University Medical School, Chicago, is doing important work. Drachman has been able to produce cognitive deficits mimicking those of senile dementia by giving normal individuals a drug, scopolamine, which is known to block the cholinergic system.

In an early study, Dr. Drachman gave nine patients with senile dementia small doses of L-dopa, a drug which is converted in the body into a neurotransmitter. Three of the nine showed pronounced intellectual improvement, two had moderate improvement, while results in the remaining four were equivocal.

A long road lies ahead, Drachman emphasizes, before it may be possible to restore failing mental powers by such treatment, but the findings suggest that there may be promise in this direction.

Meanwhile, evidence that an infectious agent, such as a slow-acting virus, may be involved in causing Alzheimer's has been gathered by other investigators.

At the University of Chicago, Dr. Sidney Schulman has transmitted a rare form of dementia, Creutzfeldt-Jakob disease, from a human patient to a rhesus monkey. He inoculated the monkey in November 1968 with brain biopsy tissue from a patient who later died of the disease, which is always fatal. In July 1974, almost six years later, the monkey developed symptoms like those in human patients with the disease. When the animal died six months later, autopsy examination of the brain showed destruction of brain areas (the cerebral cortex and thalamus) identical in type to that seen in human Creutzfeldt-Jakob disease.

Along with Creutzfeldt-Jakob disease, a number of other diseases of the brain, including kuru in man, scrapie in sheep, and Aleutian mink disease—all of which take years to develop—appear to be slow-acting virus diseases.

In 1976, Dr. Daniel Carleton Gajdusek of the National Institute of Neurological and Communicative Disorders and Stroke received the Nobel Prize for studies including those on kuru. He showed that kuru was transmitted among the native Fore people of New Guinea by the ritual eating of the brains of deceased relatives. Dr. Gajdusek and a co-worker, Dr. Clarence Gibbs, Jr., have transmitted kuru from man to chimpanzees and several species of monkeys.

In recent studies, too, one strain of scrapie, the dementia affecting sheep, has been found to induce Alzheimer-like plaques in mice.

Conceivably, if a virus can be shown incontrovertibly to be responsible for Alzheimer's, a method of treatment or even possibly a preventive vaccine might be developed.

But Is It Alzheimer's Alone— or Really Alzheimer's at All?

As of now, there is no known treatment effective against Alzheimer's disease. But, as David Drachman and many other investigators keep emphasizing, there should be no rush to write off any case of senile dementia as hopeless, irreversible.

With painstaking diagnostic efforts, Drachman notes, often a component of dementia—a disorder that is far more treatable than Alzheimer's disease—may be found.

"Dementia is the wear and tear of living which interacts with specific diseases," Drachman noted at a recent session on dementia at a meeting of the Association for Research in Nervous and Mental Diseases. "A person who has marginally compensated for this wear and tear gets a disease which tips the scale. If you find and treat the disease it makes a big difference."

This view was shared by many others at the meeting, who also agreed that many victims of dementia have not been getting the best possible treatment.

Dr. Charles Wells of Vanderbilt University Medical School

points to three different studies in which a total of 222 patients who had been diagnosed as demented were carefully re-evaluated. Fifteen percent were found to have epilepsy and other disorders, some of which, if detected early, are reversible. About 25 percent had treatable disorders in which deterioration could be halted and in some cases improvement could be obtained. Because any hope of successful treatment lies in precise diagnosis, Wells urges thorough study to detect any endocrine gland disorders and other treatable problems that may contribute to or even cause dementia symptoms. Even when Alzheimer's is the overwhelming problem, Wells emphasizes, palliative measures may be in order: correcting nutritional deficiencies, providing physical therapy, prescribing suitable hearing aids or new eyeglasses, and others which, without affecting Alzheimer's disease, nevertheless may help overall.

Dr. Robert Katzman, chairman of neurology at Albert Einstein College of Medicine, New York, calls for re-evaluating patients diagnosed as having Alzheimer's in follow-up studies even months after initial diagnosis. For one thing, he notes, it is difficult to separate patients who suffer depression as a reaction to Alzheimer's disease from those who are really suffering from depression and not Alzheimer's.

Actually, depression often accompanies dementia. In untreatable dementia, complicating depression may be severe, accelerating progression toward total disability. Yet often its presence is overlooked when a patient is considered to have organic brain disease.

Dr. Bruce D. Snyder of the University of Minnesota School of Medicine tells of a sixty-three-year-old woman who for a year had suffered from impairment of memory and other changes to the point where her husband was afraid to leave her alone. She had "blackout" episodes during which she was incontinent. She experienced auditory hallucinations and agitation, frequent crying spells, difficulty in sleeping, and weight loss due to a poor appetite.

Although she was diagnosed as demented—and, in fact, was— she was finally also diagnosed as suffering from depression. Three weeks after she was started on antidepressant drug treatment, her mood and appetite improved and she no longer had hallucinations. Treatment for the depression did not change the organic cause of dementia, but it made a major difference in her life.

Arteriosclerosis

When arteries anywhere in the body become diseased, their inner linings encrusted, the channels through which blood can flow are diminished.

When, of course, the coronary arteries which supply the heart muscle are affected, there may be anginal chest pain or heart attack.

Cerebrovascular disease—in which arteries supplying the brain are affected—can lead to stroke. For a long time, before there was awareness of Alzheimer's disease, virtually all dementia was considered to be the result of cerebrovascular disease. No longer, although it is considered to be a prime factor in some cases and a contributing factor in others.

We will be looking in detail into the relationship between senility and cerebrovascular disease—and into promising new efforts at treatment—in Chapter 5.

4

The Pseudosenilities (Pseudodementias)

She was one of a small group of people with bizarre symptoms seen over a short period of time at the Baylor College of Medicine, Houston Department of Neurology. Until two years before, she had been a healthy and successful businesswoman, a leading real estate broker. But at that point, when she was fifty-seven, she had begun to experience irritability, anxiety, depression, episodes of senseless crying, and a failing memory. Subsequently, she went on to develop other symptoms as well: incoordination, dizzy spells, tingling and numbness of feet and hands.

She was thoroughly checked for any disorder that might possibly explain her condition. None could be found. She did, however, have one problem that needed attention even though it had no known relationship to her symptoms: a very great elevation in blood-fat levels that could be a harbinger of heart attack or stroke. Her cholesterol was 600, her triglycerides 1600.

It took a combination of diet and a medication, clofibrate, to bring her triglyceride level down to 183 and cholesterol to 217 over a period of three months. At that point, all her symptoms vanished.

In five other Baylor patients, similar symptoms—a kind of hyperlipidemic (high blood-fat level) dementia—yielded to diet alone to bring down the excessive levels.

How hyperlipidemia can produce dementialike symptoms is unknown. "But the fact that patients improve when their hyperlipidemia is treated," report the Baylor neurologists, "makes it desirable to look for this defect in all patients with dementia and treat it as soon as it's found."

Hyperlipidemia is one of the more recent, dramatic examples of how symptoms much like those of true dementia can stem from problems other than organic brain disease, problems that are very often treatable, some of them even relatively easily.

Are such pseudodementias common? It now appears that they may be surprisingly common.

Many recent studies suggest that dementia often has been overdiagnosed and pseudodementia overlooked.

In a 1975 study of diagnoses of patients over the age of sixty-five in three cities, organic brain disorders were found to be diagnosed with more than 50 percent greater frequency in New York than in either London or Toronto. It's possible, of course, that the patients in the three cities differ. But it's more likely, as Dr. Charles E. Wells of Vanderbilt University has reported, "that the figures indicate that in New York elderly patients with affective [emotional] disorders were labeled as demented, whereas in Great Britain where . . . the importance of recognizing functional disorders in the aged [has been emphasized] patients with affective disorders were more likely to be labeled correctly."

But even in Great Britain, misdiagnoses are hardly unknown. Also in 1975, investigators reported on a follow-up of thirty-five patients diagnosed as having dementia at Guy's Hospital in London. The initial diagnosis was actually confirmed by progressive deterioration in only fifteen of the thirty-five.

In another British study, when 106 consecutive patients, all of whom had been screened by a neurologist or a psychologist or even by both, were hospitalized for thorough investigation of their "dementia," that diagnosis could not be corroborated in nineteen. And specific functional disorders, mostly depression, were identified in ten.

The conclusion is inescapable that diagnostic errors are not rare, observes Dr. Wells, "even when the patients are evaluated carefully by well-trained psychiatrists and neurologists."

Here in the United States in 1977, *The New Physician,* a professional journal for medical school students and young physicians just entering practice, had this report to make:

"Sophie E., 73, is confused, disoriented, frightened. Although she was alert and independent just days before, her physician settles on a diagnosis of chronic irreversible brain syndrome, a progressive disease that takes years to develop. The viral infection that caused Sophie's bout of confusion is never discovered, and she is admitted to a nursing home.

"Max H., 86, also is confused and disoriented. His physician tells Max's family that such behavior is to be expected in a man of his advanced years. He never realizes that Max has suffered a heart attack—without the chest pains, shortness of breath and other classic symptoms of myocardial infarction [heart attack].

"Jean S., 75, complains of malaise and appears confused when she appears for a regular physical. Her physician sends her home with a prescription for a tranquilizer and assurance that a woman of her age shouldn't expect "to feel like a spring chicken." But Jean's symptoms are due, not to age, but to appendicitis, again without such classic symptoms as abdominal tenderness, fever, and a high white blood count.

"The tragedy of health care for the aged is that doctors in this country often don't know what signs and symptoms to look for in their elderly patients. The reason they don't know is simple: no one ever told them." *The New Physician* added that, finally, medicine's ignorance of and indifference to geriatric care are being challenged and changed.

That older people can have underlying physical disorders which account for dementia without presenting any of the classical symptoms of those disorders has been underscored recently by Dr. Maurice H. Charlton of the University of Rochester. "For example, a patient harboring a subdural hematoma [a tumorlike mass of clotted blood between the tough casing and the more delicate membranes covering the tissue of the brain due to an injury such as a fall] need not present a history of significant head trauma or show a markedly depressed sensorium [consciousness]; subtle intellectual or aphasic defects [disturbances in comprehending or expressing speech concepts] may be the only symptoms. Similarly, hypothyroidism or vitamin B_{12} deficiency may appear primarily as dementia, without the signs and symptoms given in classical descriptions."

Says Dr. William Reichel of Baltimore, a specialist in problems of older people and former president of the American Geriatrics Society: "Because of the compromises in brain function that accompany aging, elderly patients tend to show confusion and disorientation as a first sign of infection, pneumonia, cardiac failure, coronary occlusion, electrolyte imbalance, anemia, or dehydration. The brain changes may have no behavioral expression at all in the absence of major stress. The presumption of senility or 'chronic brain syndrome' is unwarranted in the context of sudden behavioral change; rather, we may be dealing with the behavioral concomitants of a reversible medical illness or drug toxicity."

Dr. Reichel has reported the case of a sixty-six-year-old woman who was hospitalized after several days of worsening confusion and disorientation, weakness, depression, and nausea. "She was found to have the following daily drug intake: tolbutamide, methenamine mandelate, spironolactone, phenformin hydrochloride, furosemide, nitrofurantoin, and prochlorperazine [a motley assortment of agents for diabetes, edema, infection, high blood pressure, and gastrointestinal disorders]. All drugs were withdrawn. She received intravenous fluids. On discharge to her home, she showed no need for any of the drugs. Her confusion had disappeared completely."

Reactions to drugs in the elderly is, in fact, a common cause of dementia-mimicking behavioral disturbances. Older people are especially prone to adverse reactions from some drugs—particularly tranquilizers, digoxin, and diuretics—at doses generally safe in younger adults. Because of changes in body metabolism, nervous system responsiveness, and lower rates of drug elimination due to diminished kidney and liver function, drugs can have greater effect. We will be considering drug-induced pseudosenilities in more detail in Chapter 10.

Alcohol, too, especially when used in combination with drugs, can be a significant pseudosenility factor.

Say Drs. J. C. Hoogerbeets and John LaWall of the University of Arizona School of Medicine, Tucson: "In our experience, it is not uncommon to find that the patient has been taking excessive amounts of alcohol for a long time, often disguised as nightcaps. Especially when done in combination with use of certain analgesics, sedatives, and minor tranquilizers, this can lead to periodic confusional states and even to chronic confusion. Simple restriction of the use of these agents often has an immediate and dramatic effect."

Depression is another common reason for pseudodementia. "Many deteriorated elderly patients do not suffer from senile organic brain disease, but from a depression," says Dr. T. L. Brink of the San Mateo County Mental Health Department, California. "The depressed patient loses interest in his environment and may exhibit the senile's symptoms. The effects are so similar that many physicians and psychologists have difficulty in distinguishing between the two syndromes." In cases of depression (see Chapter 9), suitable treatment can produce a remission of the depression and what Brink terms "its senility-mocking symptoms."

The Hydrocephalus Pseudodementia

We began this chapter with an account of one newly recognized cause of pseudodementia—hyperlipidemia. There has been another relatively recent and no less dramatic discovery.

The patient was a man who had been a successful professional and whose problems came to a head when he was in his mid-sixties. Even ten years earlier, both he and his family had begun to note some changes in his personality. He had always been mild-mannered, slow to anger. Progressively, he became quick-tempered, argumentative, belligerent. In his early sixties, he began to experience gait disturbances, repeatedly losing his balance and falling.

Finally, his deterioration became so pronounced that he was hospitalized. He was then experiencing severe headaches, memory deficits, disorientation, and could walk no more than a few steps without falling.

The diagnosis: hydrocephalus—"water on the brain." The treatment: a surgical procedure similar to that used when a child has hydrocephalus. The result: disappearance of symptoms within days.

That hydrocephalus can be present in an older person and produce what seems like senile dementia without any of the obvious signs such as head enlargement seen in a baby was established only in 1965, when a Harvard team reported on a small series of patients with the previously unrecognized condition.

Within the brain are four reservoirs, called ventricles, which contain fluid. The ventricles, in effect, allow the brain to float on and in fluid so that shocks are absorbed.

The spinal cord, which like the brain is part of the central nervous system, also has fluid to cushion it from shock.

Normally, about half a quart of fluid is produced daily within the ventricles. It flows out through openings in the brain and arrives in the fluid cushion surrounding the spinal cord. Along with routine flow there is also routine absorption of the fluid by large veins in membranes covering the brain so the new fluid formation is balanced by the absorption.

In a hydrocephalic child, a congenital malformation prevents normal fluid flow. As a result, pressure within the ventricles increases, the ventricles become distended, and the distention makes the child's still-soft skull bones spread so that the head begins to balloon grotesquely. In most cases, hydrocephalus becomes apparent shortly after birth or during infancy, and if unchecked by early childhood it may lead to mental and physical deterioration as well as massive head enlargement.

For a hydrocephalic child, surgery is performed to divert the excess fluid. Through a small incision in the scalp and a burr hole in the skull, a fine spaghetti-thin tube is inserted into a fluid-dilated ventricle. The tube is then threaded under the scalp and under the skin of the neck to the jugular vein and down through that vein to an entrance chamber of the heart. The procedure—known as a ventriculoatrial shunt—lets the fluid flow harmlessly into the blood circulation and works wonders for a hydrocephalic child.

In an elderly person, hydrocephalus does not produce any obvious signs—no head enlargement, not even increased pressure. The first report from the Harvard team—headed by Drs. R. D. Adams, C. M. Fisher, and S. Hakim—in 1965 was surprising because it described hydrocephalus in three elderly patients with normal-size heads and normal pressure within the brain.

One was a sixty-three-year-old woman who experienced a peculiar episode of weakness, giddiness, and pallor. Although she recovered the following day, thereafter she became easily tired, uncertain of gait, forgetful, less able to concentrate and organize her daily affairs. Several times she lost urinary control.

Six months after onset of her illness, she entered Massachusetts General Hospital, a Harvard teaching hospital in Boston. There, many studies were performed, including a check for cerebrospinal fluid pressure and another in which her skull was x-rayed. Both tests were normal. But a pneumoencephalogram—an x ray of the brain after injection of air—showed massive enlargement of the ventricle system.

Very soon after a shunt operation done much as for a child with hydrocephalus, she began to improve and continued to improve. At age sixty-six, her intellectual performance in standard tests was "superior" and her general memory "very superior."

The other two patients also made dramatic recoveries after shunting. Within a month, both were judged by their families to be their former selves. One, a sixty-two-year-old pediatrician who had shown symptoms of senility, including forgetfulness, unsteady gait, and bedwetting, could return to his medical practice in excellent health.

The original Harvard work has been confirmed at many medical centers. And detection of the problem—variously called occult hydrocephalus and normal pressure hydrocephalus—is being aided now by refined diagnostic techniques including CAT (computerized axial tomography) scans.

CAT scanning is a new technique in which information is obtained with a special x-ray beam that shoots out to 160 or more different areas of the brain. The reflections are processed by a computer which turns out a picture. Unlike conventional x-ray devices that provide only two-dimensional pictures, the CAT scanner provides three-dimensional ones that reveal details and data never before available.

Normal pressure hydrocephalus is characterized by a triad that includes progressive dementia; a spastic, ataxic gait in which the feet appear to be magnetized to the floor, making it difficult to initiate movement from a standing position; and urinary incontinence.

To the triad may be added other symptoms. Victims often are slow and withdrawn, although paranoid and aggressive behavior occurs in some. Depression is frequent and sometimes severe. Drs. Harold Rosen of the Veterans Administration Hospital, Philadelphia, and Mary E. Swigar of Yale University School of Medicine have recently found that the early course of normal pressure hydrocephalus may sometimes be characterized by symptoms of apathy, inattentiveness, agitation, and poverty of thought, which mimick a depressive illness.

What causes the hydrocephalus? In about two-thirds of cases, it appears to be the result of brain injury, hemorrhage, infection, or tumors. In the remaining cases, no cause has been identified.

The shunting operation is neither a panacea nor a minor procedure. As with any surgery, there is some risk of infection and other possible complications. But it is clearly a worthwhile procedure when appropriately used for patients who might otherwise have a hopeless outlook.

Results are not always predictable. It can produce dramatic reversal of symptoms in some cases; in others it may stop progression of illness.

Overall, improvement has been reported in about 55 percent of patients, with better results (65 percent improved) in those in whom the hydrocephalus is linked to a known cause than in others (41 percent improved).

Other Causes

It has become apparent that there are scores of possible causes for pseudodementia—remediable causes.

Glandular problems—notably those of the thyroid—can be responsible. In one case, for example, a seventy-year-old woman suffered a striking memory loss and intellectual decline over a period of a year. When finally she was studied thoroughly, she was found to have hypothyroidism—underfunctioning of the thyroid gland. Several months of thyroid extract treatment to make up for the deficiency improved her memory and intellectual function to what they had been years before.

When a weakened heart is treated so that its pumping efficiency is restored and blood flow to the brain as well as other body areas is improved, confusion and other symptoms may disappear.

Correct an anemia, which impairs the oxygen-carrying capacity of the blood, and mentation may improve.

It may improve, too, when a nutritional deficiency is corrected. When a seventy-two-year-old woman was finally hospitalized for thorough study because of confusion and failing physical health after her physician had been unable to offer much help, she was found to have previously unsuspected pellagra, caused by a deficiency of the vitamin niacin. Within a few weeks after niacin treatment began, her physical symptoms vanished and her confusion cleared.

We will be considering these and other problems as well that can lead to pseudosenility—and how they can be overcome.

Their recognition and treatment can help rescue many of the elderly who may be suffering needlessly and may be looked upon as hopelessly senile when they are not; some are preventable problems and their prevention by suitable, often simple measures can help to assure avoidance of senility.

5

When It's a Matter of Brain Circulation

At a 1976 joint meeting on stroke and cerebral circulation held in Dallas, Dr. Gary G. Ferguson, assistant professor of neurosurgery at University Hospital, London, Ontario, reported on a group of ten patients with dementia associated with disease of arteries in the neck leading to the brain.

The average age of the patients, all of whom were men, was sixty years. The average period of dementia was six months. Two patients had shown symptoms for more than two years.

In addition to the symptoms of dementia, all had manifested signs of cerebrovascular disease such as "little strokes"—fleeting episodes of stumbling, numbness or paralysis of fingers of one hand, vision blurring, or loss of speech or memory.

Examination had revealed that all had multiple "extracranial occlusive disease"—narrowing and blockage of several arteries in the neck area supplying blood to the brain. In three of the patients, four vessels—the internal carotid artery on each side and the vertebral artery on each side—had been affected. In five, the two carotids had been occluded or closed off. And two had a miscellaneous collection of narrowings and blockages.

In an attempt to overcome the reduction in brain blood flow resulting from the occlusions, surgery was carried out, bypassing the blockages by connecting up healthy vessels.

41

All of the patients had been severely disabled before operation. None had been able to work; two had been institutionalized. Postoperatively, five patients were "dramatically improved"—two who had shown signs of dementia for more than two years returned to work, while the other three were able to work on a limited basis. Of the remaining five, four showed some improvement as judged by their families, while one failed to improve at all.

"It's a rare combination," Dr. Ferguson reported, "but there is no doubt some patients with dementia also have severe occlusive cerebrovascular disease in the neck, and I think it's reasonable to propose a relationship between the two."

A few months after Dr. Ferguson gave his report, Dr. C. Doyle Haynes, clinical associate professor of surgery at Emory University School of Medicine, Atlanta, had another to make at a meeting of the Society of Vascular Surgery in Albuquerque.

Carotid endarterectomy is a procedure often used now to try to prevent massive stroke in patients experiencing little-stroke symptoms because of blockage of a carotid artery in the neck. It involves opening up the artery at a point where special x-ray studies have shown blockage and then reaming out the blocking material and closing the artery up again.

What Haynes had to report was that quite possibly carotid endarterectomy may do more than prevent major strokes—that it may improve a patient's mental abilities, at least insofar as these are measured by IQ and other psychological tests.

Haynes's clinical impression that such improvement might occur was based on casual observations he had made of many patients undergoing endarterectomy. He was aware, too, of observations by others that endarterectomy might improve a patient's mental status. In fact, some studies of this had been made, but they lacked controls—comparable patients not undergoing surgery with whom comparisons could be made.

Haynes used as controls a group of patients scheduled to undergo surgery unrelated to cerebral blood flow, in whom no particular change in mental ability was to be expected, and who could be matched with endarterectomy patients for age, sex, education, and race.

With the help of psychologists from Auburn University, the preoperative and postoperative performances of seventeen endarterectomy patients and eight other surgical patients were compared. Patients in both groups took psychological tests within twenty-four hours before their operations and again four and eight weeks afterward. The tests included a shortened version of the standard Wechsler Adult Intelligence Scale, the Minnesota Multiphasic Personality Inventory, the State-Trait Anxiety Inventory, and a "trails test" in which the subject connects randomly placed numbered circles in their correct sequence as fast as he can.

It turned out that the endarterectomy patients had less "trait anxiety"—meaning chronic predisposition to feeling anxious—after surgery than before, while the control patients showed no differences.

Other interesting changes measured by the Minnesota Multiphasic Personality Inventory turned up only in the endarterectomy group. These patients had lower postoperative scores for confusion, disorientation, and suspicion.

Endarterectomy patients after surgery also did better on the trails tests. There is an "easy" and a "hard" version. Before surgery, the endarterectomy patients averaged 112.2 seconds for the easier test, compared with 51.4 seconds for the control patients. After surgery, the endarterectomy group reduced the average time to 70.4 seconds, for a 41.8 second gain, while the control group stayed virtually steady at 53.4 seconds. On the more complicated test version, the endarterectomy patients' preoperative average was 212.7 seconds compared with the controls' 159.5 seconds. After surgery, the endarterectomy patients had an average score of 154.9 seconds, a 57.8 second improvement, while the controls actually lost ground to 176.3 seconds.

Performance on the IQ tests also was impressive. In both verbal and perceptual IQ tests, the endarterectomy patients had higher average scores after surgery, while the control patients' average scores dropped slightly. Some of the endarterectomy patients showed great improvement—as much as 22.5 points on the verbal test and as much as 35.1 points on the perceptual.

How does Haynes interpret these results? Certainly, he emphasizes, endarterectomy is not a cure for senility. "We're helping," he believes, "to alleviate symptoms of senility by increasing blood flow to the brain."

A New Perspective on Arteriosclerosis and Senility

Once it was the custom—among physicians as well as lay people—to attribute all mental decline and dementia in older people to cerebral arteriosclerosis, or hardening and narrowing of brain arteries.

That is no longer valid. Although some recent studies indicate that too many physicians may still make such an offhanded diagnosis and may still consider mental decline and dementia to be inevitable with aging, many careful investigations have established, as we have seen earlier, that more often the problem lies elsewhere.

But even authorities who emphasize the latter view acknowledge that in some cases arteriosclerosis is related to dementia through the artery disease's role in producing brain infarcts, the starvation and death of areas of brain tissue. They consider that multiple infarcts can produce a condition in which dementia is the dominant symptom, and there is a history of recurrent strokes or little strokes.

And the ability to help such people has developed as the result of some relatively recent remarkable advances in understanding the nature and course of little strokes and big strokes and in techniques of correcting the former in order to help minimize the risk of the latter.

Strokes and Little Strokes

Each year in the United States, stroke affects 500,000 people, most of them elderly but some in their forties, and claims at least 200,000 lives.

Also known as apoplexy and cerebrovascular accident (CVA), stroke until recently was regarded with such fatalism that little was done to try to prevent it or its end results.

A stroke is the result of disease of arteries in or leading to the brain. In some cases, an artery may leak or burst, resulting in hemorrhage into the brain substance. In most cases, an artery becomes obstructed.

Since a stroke may result from disease in a large or small artery anywhere in the brain or leading to it, the consequences can be varied. A stroke may block out a tiny area of the memory center or may deprive a large section of brain of oxygen, producing unconsciousness, paralysis, labored breathing and death.

One of the first important modern developments was the discovery that a fairly substantial number of strokes stem from damage to arteries outside the brain, in the neck, where they are accessible to surgical repair.

Another—and related—development was the recognition that while a major stroke may seem to strike suddenly, the stroke process is not sudden, and commonly may provide early warning signals—little strokes.

Also known as transient ischemic attacks (TIA's)—ischemic meaning related to blood deficiency—little strokes can produce a great variety of symptoms.

The warning symptoms. A little stroke may bring sudden visual loss in one eye—"like a shade coming down"—that partially or completely obscures the vision field. The denseness of the loss can vary, from a "graying out" or "looking through rain on a window" effect to total blindness. The duration usually is short, about five minutes, and recovery is nearly always complete.

There may be transient weakness or heaviness of an arm or

leg, and often arm weakness is accompanied by facial weakness.

Tingling, "pins and needles," or numbness in limbs or face may occur, usually lasting no more than thirty minutes and accompanied by weakness.

There may be speech disturbances along with difficulties in reading or writing, and, rarely, fleeting confusional states. Vertigo may occur, accompanied by unsteadiness, and walking as though drunk.

Visual disturbances other than those already described may occur: upsets in both eyes, with bizarre shapes, patterns, colors, flashes, and lines—and sometimes double vision.

In some cases, "drop" attacks may occur—falls without warning with only brief loss of consciousness.

If a patient with any of these symptoms heeds them and seeks medical help, diagnostic techniques such as special x rays of the arteries leading to the brain can be used to determine if there is an obstruction that can be reached.

If so, under either general or local anesthesia, an incision several inches long can be made along the side of the neck. The affected section of artery is then opened and clogging deposits are reamed out, opening up the channel for increased blood flow. In some cases, a bypass graft may be used, providing blood with a new channel to flow through around the obstructed area.

After such surgery, pain is moderate, relieved readily, and the patient may be up and moving about the following day or even the same day. Recovery is speedy, often requiring only a few days.

New Surgery

Much more recently has come a major new surgical development, a way to do the seemingly impossible: help many patients who have obstructions in the smaller arteries buried within the brain.

It had to wait for the development of remarkable microinstrumentation: extremely tiny scissors, probes, hooks, blood vessel clips, suture-needle holders, and sutures of nylon only twenty micrometers in diameter (one-fourth the thickness of a human hair) with which to join vessels only about 1/25th of an inch in diameter.

In the new procedure, called cerebral revascularization, a segment of an artery that supplies blood to the scalp (the superficial temporal artery) is joined, through an opening made in the skull, to a segment of the middle cerebral artery which extends over the brain surface. This creates a bypass of the circulation beyond a blockage and connects two arteries which are rarely affected by disease. Since the scalp has a rich blood supply, it can spare the superficial temporal artery.

Today, surgeons at the New York University Medical Center, at Albert Einstein College of Medicine in the Bronx, at the University of Minnesota, Minneapolis, and at an increasing number of medical centers are performing the procedure.

Reporting on the first patients to be operated on at Albert Einstein, Dr. Jack M. Fein noted that "of some 30 patients operated on by our group only one has subsequently had a stroke, and that was related to a pulmonary embolism [a blood clot in a lung] a month after surgery. We have not had a single procedure-related death."

At an international symposium in which results in 400 patients treated at various centers were reported after a follow-up time averaging two and a half years, only three had suffered a stroke, and there was a significant reduction in the frequency of little-stroke episodes for all patients who had previously experienced them, with the episodes completely eliminated in most.

Promising Non-Surgical Developments

Not by any means has all the progress been made by surgeons.

High blood pressure plays a significant role in strokes, as has become evident from a whole series of studies, including the government's famed long-term Framingham Study which has followed some 5000 originally healthy people in that Massachusetts community since 1949. We will be discussing such studies in detail later, and other studies as well which show the value of controlling high blood pressure for reducing the risk of stroke. Also to be discussed later: other clearly established risk factors for both stroke and heart attacks and the effects of countering them.

Very recently, too, has come recognition of the role of certain blood elements, called platelets, in strokes and heart attacks; and with that recognition came trials with already promising results of measures to counter dangerous platelet activity.

Platelets are tiny disklike bodies in the blood with an important role to play in forming blood clots to prevent hemorrhaging when a blood vessel is broken.

But recent studies have shown that platelets may clump together and form aggregates at narrowed areas in blood vessels and, in doing so, may block flow and initiate strokes. Such abnormal platelet activity has been found in people experiencing little strokes and in those with the anginal chest pain of heart disease as well.

At the same time, some drugs—already available ones—have proved to have the power to stop abnormal platelet clumping. One is aspirin. Another is Anturane, a medication long used to treat gouty arthritis. A third is Persantine, which has been used for relieving anginal pain.

Already, there have been promising results with aspirin, and trials with the other drugs are under way. (Anturane has already been found to halve the sudden death rate in people who have had a heart attack.)

In a recent thirty-seven-month period at ten major U.S. medical centers, daily aspirin strikingly improved the outlook for little-stroke patients. Of patients receiving four aspirins a day, 88 percent either had no additional little strokes or a significantly reduced number.

Other studies have been carried out with aspirin at Baylor College of Medicine, Houston, and in Canada. In the Canadian trial in twelve medical centers with 585 little-stroke patients, lasting from November 1971 through June 1977, patients receiving four aspirins a day had, overall, a one-third lower incidence of major strokes and death. Among the men in the trial, the reduction approached 50 percent; and why they should benefit more than women remains to be explained.

In the Texas trial, patients included not only those with little strokes but others who had already suffered a major stroke. And four aspirins a day benefited both groups. "Aspirin appears to be very helpful to patients at risk of major stroke," reports Dr. John S. Meyer of Baylor. "It can be used early on in the disease process when vigorous treatment is important. It also seems to help reverse the disease process among patients who have had a major stroke."

Other Little-Stroke Factors

Other factors have been found to provoke little-stroke episodes. They include disordered heart rhythms, congestive heart failure, even anemia—all of which we will consider later.

Vasodilator Drugs

A considerable amount of debate is taking place among investigators over the value of certain drugs called vasodilators in combating dementia.

Vasodilators are agents that may dilate narrowed blood vessels. They are often prescribed for patients who show senile mental changes which may be related to reduced blood circulation to the brain.

The physiologic effects of one widely used vasodilator, cyclandelate, have been well documented. The drug is effective in dilating arteries of the skull and brain and in increasing the volume of circulating blood in patients with cerebrovascular disease.

Its efficacy in providing relief of symptoms, however, has not been documented so clearly. Some investigators have reported good results, others have reported equivocal or negative results.

Feeling that vasodilators in the past have too often been prescribed indiscriminately, without proper selection of patients, a group of physicians headed by Dr. D. B. Rao, all of the Department of Medicine in Geriatrics and Chronic Diseases of Oak Forest (Illinois) Hospital, recently undertook a study of the efficacy of cyclandelate for symptoms of senility, under scientifically controlled conditions.

Sixty men and women aged sixty-five or older were selected for the study. All had clearly evident symptoms of senility. No patient with a history of Alzheimer's disease, psychiatric illness, or with debility so severe as to make the possibility of significant improvement unlikely was included.

The patients were randomly assigned to either of two groups, those in one receiving 1600 milligrams of cyclandelate daily while those in the other received the same dosage of an identical-appearing but inert preparation (placebo).

The study went on for twelve weeks, and at the beginning and each four weeks thereafter the patients were examined physically and were also evaluated with several standard psychologic scales.

Among the factors that were evaluated were confusion, mental alertness, impairment of recent memory, mood depression, self-care, emotional disability, anxiety, instability, indifference to surroundings, unsociability, uncooperativeness, bothersomeness, and hostility.

At the conclusion of the study, the investigators found cyclandelate to be significantly more effective than placebos in improving all of these factors. The positive effect of cyclandelate on impairment of recent memory, mood depression, irritability, hostility, indifference to surroundings, and anxiety was significantly superior to that of placebos as early as the eighth week of treatment.

The investigators concluded: "The clinical evidence suggests that prudent use of cerebral vasodilators such as cyclandelate may definitely delay senile deterioration."

Hydergine is another vasodilator which has been used extensively—but not always with clear-cut results. Some investigators have reported no significant changes; others have reported improvements in a small proportion of patients. A number of studies have compared Hydergine and placebos; in these, the particular symptoms that responded varied from one investigation to another. For example, in one study Hydergine was found to produce significant improvement of physical manifestations of senility and in daily living activities but did not affect psychological status. Another reported significant improvement in attitude and mood, and still another found improvement in cognition and intellectual function.

In one of the most recent studies, carried out by Dr. Charles M. Gaitz and other investigators of the Texas Research Institute of Mental Sciences, Houston, and the University of Texas Medical Branch, Galveston, fifty-four elderly male and female nursing home residents participated. All had apparent and persistent cognitive, emotional, and physical symptoms associated with senile mental deterioration.

This, too, was a study using an active drug for some patients and placebos for others to provide a basis for comparison. An eighteen-category symptom rating scale was used for periodic assessment over a six-month interval. Comparison of the two groups of patients showed significantly more improvement among the Hydergine-treated, especially during the last three months of treatment, in such factors as confusion, mental alertness, impairment of recent memory, and mood depression.

It's the conviction of many leading investigators that while vasodilators are far from being panaceas—and, too, while it is difficult if not impossible to forecast in advance whether a particular patient may benefit—they do bring about some degree of improvement, sometimes quite worthwhile improvement, in some patients when used for at least two months or longer.

There is another aspect to the vasodilator picture. There has been evidence that when benefits have occurred from use of the drugs, they have not always correlated well with increased blood flow. It now appears that all vasodilators are not alike and that dilation in fact may be only one effect and not necessarily the prime effect of some. There are indications, for example, that some may improve the brain's use of oxygen and nutrients.

Newer drugs of the vasodilator class are being developed and studied (see Chapter 15) with the hope they may have definable effects that could make them useful for more patients.

A Psychochemical Approach

Dr. Arthur C. Walsh of the University of Pittsburgh for some years has been experimenting, with reported success, in using a combination of anticoagulant treatment and psychotherapy to help patients with senile and presenile dementia.

Walsh, a psychiatrist, developed his approach to treatment after becoming intrigued with the work of Dr. M. H. Knisely of the Medical University of South Carolina. Knisely reported that as narrowing of arteries occurs and slows blood flow, something else happens. The slowing leads to a reduction of certain normal forces and this allows red blood cells to sludge, adhering to each other and forming aggregations which impair blood flow further.

Knisely also found that diabetes and alcoholism, among other conditions, can cause blood sludging—which, as Walsh notes, could account for why brain damage is more common among people with these conditions.

Anticoagulants are drugs that inhibit blood clotting, tending to maintain the blood in a fluid state. In an early study, Walsh worked with a group of fifteen alcohol-brain-damaged patients. After many other treatment methods had failed, twelve of the fifteen responded to anticoagulant therapy.

The first patient with symptoms of senile dementia to receive the treatment was a sixty-three-year-old woman who had deteriorated steadily over a three-year period. She no longer could use the bathroom, dress herself, or light her own cigarette.

She was given an anticoagulant, Dicumarol. After two months on the drug, she showed noteworthy improvement. In addition to becoming able to take care of herself and carry out her own personal hygiene, she managed now to do meticulous needlework again. She continued on the drug during the remaining eighteen months of her life, living by herself most of the time and even doing some of her own interior decorating, before she suffered a fatal heart attack.

Of the next thirteen patients to receive Dicumarol, none deteriorated while on the drug, three became able to feed themselves, and one became well enough to be discharged.

Walsh then went on to another trial in which he coupled brief but intensive psychotherapy with Dicumarol treatment. Twenty-two patients took part. They ranged up to eighty-nine years of age; most had symptoms of disorientation, impaired memory, poor judgment, loss of intellectual ability; eight suffered mainly from anxiety, depression, or paranoid ideas.

The objective of psychotherapy was to get patients to express feelings of fear, frustration, persecution, abandonment. Once exposed, the feelings could be discussed in order to reduce stress to a minimum. If improvement occurred over a two-month period, patients were referred to their own physicians for maintenance therapy.

All twenty-two showed some degree of improvement by the end of two months. In eight, the improvement was marked. In fourteen, results were classified as good: memory considerably improved, confusion greatly reduced or eliminated.

At a recent American Psychiatric Association meeting, Walsh presented the findings of his latest study with forty-nine patients, many of whom were extremely deteriorated and nearly all of whom had been treated unsuccessfully elsewhere.

By now, he had switched to another anticoagulant, Coumadin (sodium warfarin), which he found easier to control than Dicumarol, and use of which for other purposes is familiar to most doctors.

Placed on individualized daily doses of the anticoagulant and provided with individual and family psychotherapy, Walsh reported, 70 percent of these otherwise hopeless patients improved, 15 percent dramatically. Two patients had no change; nine got worse; and four died of various causes.

In his report, Walsh gave as an example of marked improvement the case of an eighty-one-year-old Ohio woman, diagnosed as senile, who could not sign her name prior to treatment and was so weak she had to be hospitalized. In the hospital, she lay in her bed, staring blankly at the wall, fervently clutching a stuffed dog.

Several weeks later, on treatment, "she wrote a note of gratitude in her own handwriting and was able to discuss her illness and other problems very sensibly."

Anticoagulant treatment is not without risk. Whenever it is used, it must be used carefully, under close medical supervision, for an excessive dose can lead to hemorrhaging.

Walsh acknowledges that "there is no guarantee of a good result and there is some risk of serious complications and even death." But, he emphasizes, "the majority of patients do improve significantly."

He adds that "As in other diseases, the earlier the treatment, the better the result." But, he notes, he has seen reversals in "hopeless" older patients. "Surprisingly, some of the very bad patients—several so deteriorated that we hesitated treating them—did better than others who seemed to have a better prognosis."

Improvement, Walsh reports, usually begins from four or five weeks to four months after treatment. If improvement occurs, he recommends continued anticoagulant use. In his experience, half of patients who improve regress when taken off anticoagulant treatment.

6

The Heart, the Blood, and the Mind

Few bother to distinguish among the many interesting diseases of old age and the wastebasket diagnosis of . . . senility. . . . When we throw open the shutters of our minds, permitting renewed interest and new knowledge to illuminate our thinking, we find a veritable treasure-trove of fascinating abnormal and reversible conditions among aged patients.

—Raymond Harris, M.D., Albany Medical College

It need not be a blocked blood vessel. Any condition that interferes with normal flow of blood to the brain or with the oxygen-richness of that blood can be involved.

If this were widely enough realized—among physicians as well as public—much mental deterioration as well as physical suffering could be avoided or overcome.

What are the conditions?

They include:

- Congestive heart failure—not necessarily as formidable as it sounds;
- Heart rhythm abnormalities—also not necessarily grave;
- Anemia—common, often neglected;
- Polycythemia—the reverse of anemia;
- Inflammatory artery disease—often readily controllable.

CONGESTIVE HEART FAILURE

It has an ominous ring, as if it represented a final, hopeless state of heart disease. It does not mean that at all. What it does mean is that the pumping performance of the heart is impaired and blood circulation to body tissues is reduced.

A common early symptom is gradual loss of energy over a period of months or even years. Shortness of breath on exertion may develop. There may be wheezing and nonproductive coughing. As the failure advances, there may be palpitation, sweating, and in some cases fainting. And, with progression, there is loss of mental vigor, memory suffers, and judgment becomes impaired.

What happens to produce these symptoms?

Normally, the heart has great reserve power. At rest, it uses as little as one-fourth of its actual capacity. When necessary, with strenuous physical activity, for example, it can quadruple its effort. It is normal for heart muscle fibers to grow in size to meet the needs of people who do heavy work.

Even with heavy work or vigorous athletic activity, the demands on the heart are far from excessive. If, for example, you are an office worker or have another sedentary job, there will be times during the day when you are more active than at other times, and during those periods of greater activity, the work load on the heart may average about 150 percent of the resting work load. A laborer doing heavy physical work may impose an average 200 percent work load on his heart over a twenty-four-hour period.

But when an abnormal condition affects the heart, the work load can be much greater. With severely elevated blood pressure, for example, the work load on the heart may be doubled for twenty-four hours a day.

As the heart is subjected to extra demands by high blood pressure or other disease, it responds by increasing in size and weight. For a time—months to years—it does well. But then it begins to falter. Heart muscle fibers, long overextended, begin to lose their strength, somewhat in the fashion of an overstretched spring. At this point, the heart contracts less vigorously, less blood is pumped out to the body, the heart may not completely empty, and pressure builds up within the heart.

The pressure may be transmitted back to the lungs through the pulmonary vein which brings blood from the lungs to the heart. With that, more blood tends to accumulate in the lungs, which then become heavier and stiffer, causing some shortness of breath.

And with less blood pumped to the body, the kidneys get less, with some impairment of their function and a drop in urine output. That means retention of more water in the blood, which increases the volume of blood and adds to lung congestion.

Pressure also may extend backward from the heart to the vein system of the body, so that less blood returns to the heart and fluid accumulates in body tissues, swelling ankles and abdomen.

And, with reduction of blood flow to the brain, there may be chronic irritability, decreased mental performance, and other symptoms.

Treatment

Congestive heart failure commonly responds to vigorous treatment.

There are three objectives of such treatment: to improve heart pumping efficiency; eliminate excess fluids; and reduce the overload on the heart by bed rest if necessary and, where possible, by treatment of the condition that led to failure.

To improve pumping efficiency, the drug digitalis is often used. More than two centuries old, it remains a mainstay of therapy. In effect, digitalis acts as a heart tonic, strengthening heart muscle fibers and increasing the force of contraction. The improvement in performance may be enough so that even if the underlying cause of failure cannot be corrected, the heart may function effectively. Often, even when failure is advanced, digitalis therapy may lead to a loss of twenty pounds of fluids from lungs, abdomen, and elsewhere.

Digitalis treatment must be individualized. When doses are too small, they do little good. But excessive doses can lead to heart rhythm disturbances, nausea, vomiting, diarrhea, headache, lethargy, and other symptoms.

Other measures may be used to eliminate excess fluids. Reducing salt intake can be important. Once, before the era of modern diuretic drugs (see below), it was necessary to severely restrict salt in the diet because salt tends to hold water in the body. Now it is usually possible for a patient to get along well without special salt-free foods, simply by using regular foods and not adding salt during preparation or at the table.

Diuretic drugs, which act to rid the body of excess fluids, are valuable for congestive heart failure and, at the same time, are useful for lowering high blood pressure when that is present.

Causes

Congestive heart failure is not a disease in itself but rather a complex of symptoms that can stem from varied causes.

A common cause is high blood pressure, and we will be discussing that in some detail in Chapter 7. We will also be looking at another cause—excessive thyroid gland activity—in Chapter 8.

Here we can consider those heart problems which can lead to congestive failure.

One is pericardial disease.

The pericardium is a sac enclosing the heart. In acute pericarditis, bacteria or viruses may invade the sac and produce inflammation. The sac inflammation also may develop as a complication when the heart is inflamed by rheumatic fever or a heart attack.

Most patients recover from the acute episode during which fever and chest pain are prominent symptoms. Sometimes, acute pericarditis is accompanied by accumulation of fluid between the layers of the sac. If the fluid accumulation is sizable, it may compress the heart enough so that the flow of blood returning to the heart from the body is impeded. In such cases, the removal of fluid brings relief. A needle is inserted through the chest wall into the pericardial sac and the fluid is withdrawn. The procedure, which is not as formidable as it sounds, is usually carried out by a heart surgeon who, by following changes on an electrocardiogram, can tell when he has reached the right area for fluid withdrawal.

Sometimes the problem lies with chronic constrictive pericarditis, in which the pericardial sac becomes abnormally thickened, losing flexibility and then acting like a rigid container around the heart, interfering with heart action. The thickening may be the result of tuberculosis; occasionally bacterial or viral pericarditis may produce it.

Treatment is surgical. The operation—pericardiectomy—was actually the first elective surgical procedure to be performed on the heart and was a milestone in modern heart surgery. In the operation, the constricting sac is removed. Afterward, the patient is greatly improved.

Congestive heart failure may also be triggered by rheumatic heart disease. In such disease, which may follow rheumatic fever, a heart valve is affected. Most commonly, the mitral valve becomes stenosed, or unable to open properly. The valve controls movement of blood into the heart chamber from which it is pumped to the body. Mitral stenosis impairs blood circulation to the body.

Says Dr. Kenneth B. Lewis of Johns Hopkins University, Baltimore: "While the incidence of acute rheumatic fever in childhood has declined dramatically in the past two or three decades (thanks to use of antibiotics), there is still a large reservoir of rheumatic heart disease among the adult population, and it is not confined, as is generally thought, to adults in the 30-to-50-year age group. The diagnosis has been missed in several elderly patients admitted to our hospital recently."

When properly diagnosed, mitral stenosis can be treated with surgical repair of the defective valve, possible even in patients in their seventies.

Previously undiagnosed congenital heart defects can also be a cause of congestive heart failure in older people. Although, by definition of course, a congenital defect is present at birth, it may or may not give rise to symptoms then. Many people with milder congenital heart anomalies enjoy good health for many years. Sometimes, however, problems may arise later.

One anomaly which is being detected among older people is atrial septal defect. This is an abnormal opening in the upper part of the wall, or septum, which separates the two upper chambers of the heart. It can allow fresh oxygen-rich blood coming from the lungs and entering one chamber to be sent over to the other chamber and then back again needlessly to the lungs instead of to the body. That means extra work for the heart, which after an extended period may weaken under the burden and lose pumping efficiency.

In older people as well as in children, surgery to close the defect can be totally corrective.

ABNORMAL HEART RHYTHMS

These tend to increase with age. Some studies of older people in homes for the aged indicate that as many as 35 percent have disturbances of heart rhythm.

Many are not serious, produce no symptoms, and require no treatment. But some can affect circulation to the brain and can be responsible for fainting or near-fainting, pallor, weakness, lightheadedness, and fatigue.

Evaluating an abnormal rhythm in an older patient sometimes may present problems. The patient may complain, for example, of repeated fluttering in the chest, yet when the physician sees him, the electrocardiogram is normal. In such cases, it is often helpful to have the patient wear a twenty-four-hour portable recorder to pick up intermittent abnormalities that otherwise are missed.

A special instrument is attached to the usual ECG leads taped to the chest, and the patient can carry it unobtrusively by an over-the-shoulder strap during normal activities.

Instead of being transferred directly to a piece of paper, the electrical impulses from the heart are recorded on magnetic tape in the instrument. The recording is continuous all the time the patient wears the device. Afterward, the tape recording can be played back by the physician on a scanner unit in about forty-five minutes. Should any abnormality be noticed, a regular paper recording of this portion of the tape is easily obtained.

Many medications are available for controlling various abnormal rhythms. They include quinidine, procainamide, lidocaine, Dilantin, propranolol, and isoproterenol.

Heart block is another problem that becomes more common with aging.

Normally, the heart is paced—its beat regulated—by electrical impulses originating in a collection of cells, called the sinoatrial node, in the upper right quarter of the right top chamber of the heart. The impulses travel through muscle fibers to initiate contraction of the top chambers of the heart and also to activate another bundle of cells, the atrioventricular node, in the lower left quarter of the right top chamber; and from here, through special conduction tissues, the impulses move rapidly to all parts of the lower pumping chambers of the heart.

When one or more major elements of the conduction system are disrupted, heart block of varying severity may develop. The impulses do not get through properly, and the pumping action of the heart is affected. The patient may experience episodes of giddiness, faintness, fainting, and sometimes even convulsions as the impaired pumping action diminishes blood flow to the brain.

Heart block can result from injury or disease. It can follow a heart attack even when, as frequently happens in older people, the heart attack is silent, producing none of the usual heart attack symptoms such as crushing chest pain.

Fortunately, heart block commonly can be overcome with a pacemaker—an electronic device designed to bypass the defective conduction system and keep an otherwise good heart beating and pumping at a rate to meet the patient's needs.

The first such device was used for a Swedish engineer in 1949. He was then only thirty-eight, a former hockey player; but his heart's electrical system had become defective, his heartbeat sometimes dropped to twenty-eight times a minute instead of seventy, and he often fainted from attacks that came unpredictably. With each attack, his wife or a friend—someone had to be with him constantly—had to thump his chest to keep him alive. A pacemaker has since triggered hundreds of millions of heartbeats for him, allowed him to live a normal life and even to fly around the world in connection with his work.

Since that first pacemaker, there have been many improvements. "Demand" pacemakers have become available; they contain a special circuit that senses the heart's electrical activity and starts the pacemaker operating only when it is actually needed to supplement the heart's activity and keep the beat steady; the pacemaker shuts off automatically when support is not needed.

At the beginning, pacemaker implantation required opening the chest so wires could be sewn to the surface of the heart. Now, however, transvenous pacemakers are in use. Under local anesthesia, electrodes are maneuvered into the heart through a catheter, or tube, inserted into a vein in the arm. The catheter is secured by tying it to the vein at the incision site, and the length of electrode remaining outside the vein is threaded under the skin and fatty layer to a site on the chest or abdomen where the pacemaker is sewn in place under the skin.

Pacemakers today are being implanted transvenously in patients ranging in age up through the nineties.

ANEMIA

All body tissues, especially those of the brain, require oxygen. And for that, not only must the heart pump well and blood vessels be open; blood quality is vital.

Diffusing from the lungs into the bloodstream, oxygen must be picked up and transported by hemoglobin, the pigment that gives red blood cells their color.

When, for any reason, either the number of red cells or the hemoglobin in those cells is inadequate, oxygen transport to the tissues is impaired and anemia is present.

The word anemia has been so bandied about that almost everyone knows or thinks he knows about the problem. Commonly, it is regarded as a matter of a pallid look and under-par feelings, readily overcome with vitamins or iron tablets or both.

But anemia is much more.

It wears many guises. It can, in fact, produce pallor, feelings of vague unwellness, malaise, tiredness, lack of energy—and sometimes even apathy and exhaustion.

Many other symptoms can stem from it: loss of appetite, nausea, vomiting, diarrhea, attacks of abdominal pain, tongue soreness, crawling or prickling sensations, shortness of breath, difficulty in walking, weakness and stiffness of the legs.

And it can be the reason for clouding of the mind and even psychotic behavior. If rarely a sole cause of dementia, anemia can contribute to it, and its correction may make a marked difference for someone who seems hopelessly senile.

Moreover, anemia is common—present, for example, in at least 20 percent of all patients admitted to general hospitals, no matter at what age or for what reason.

Its possible causes are many.

Red blood cells are created mainly in the marrow of short, flat bones. They function for up to 120 days and then, worn out, are removed from the circulation and destroyed in the spleen. Normally, the supply is being replenished constantly.

Hemoglobin consists of a protein called heme, which contains iron, and globin, another protein. Each red cell contains some 250 million hemoglobin molecules, each of which can pick up and transport eight atoms of oxygen.

With all the hemoglobins in each cell and the trillions of red cells normally present in the bloodstream, the blood's ability to transport oxygen is huge—on the order of more than 50 sextillion atoms (50 followed by 21 zeros) each minute.

One common reason for anemia is iron deficiency. The deficiency—which results in a low content of hemoglobin in red cells—may occur in childhood because of inadequate iron in the diet, especially when large amounts of milk are consumed to the exclusion of other foods. It is common in women through the menstrual years when iron is lost in the periodic blood flow.

And it is common in older people, often as the result of poor diet and sometimes as the result of blood loss because of internal bleeding such as from an ulcer.

The medical diagnosis of iron deficiency anemia—and of other types as well—is easily made with simple blood tests. When it is a matter of inadequate iron intake, the deficiency can be quickly corrected with a suitable iron supplement and thereafter avoided with suitable diet. Good sources of iron include meats, most green vegetables, raisins, nuts, prunes, dates, and dry beans. But if the deficiency results wholly or in part from internal bleeding, the source of bleeding must be found and corrected. A danger of indiscriminate dosing with iron preparations is that internal bleeding may be overlooked.

There are other types of anemia.

Hemolytic anemias result from excessive destruction of red

blood cells, outpacing the marrow's ability to supply replacements.

The destruction can be caused by exposure to excessive amounts of chemicals such as lead and arsenic or to poisonous materials that may be produced by some bacteria during severe infection. The anemia responds to avoidance of the chemicals or treatment to overcome the infection. Some people have an inherited anomaly of red cells that makes them sensitive to certain medications such as sulfa drugs. They may go through a lifetime without developing anemia unless they happen to take a sensitizing drug, which must then be stopped promptly.

There are other anemias in which inadequate red cell formation is the problem.

Pernicious anemia is an important one. The word pernicious is a hangover. It was originally used because this type of anemia was once mysterious and deadly.

It is caused by failure to absorb vitamin B_{12} from the intestine. The vitamin is required for bone marrow activity, and when it is lacking, red cells formed in the marrow are abnormally large, fail to divide, and have an abbreviated life span. The basic defect is a deficiency of "intrinsic factor," a material normally present in gastric juice in the stomach and required to promote absorption of the vitamin. Pernicious anemia today is readily treatable with occasional injections of vitamin B_{12} to circumvent the intrinsic factory deficiency.

Pernicious anemia deserves special consideration here—for one thing, because although it can occur at any age it most commonly affects people over fifty. For another, it can provoke a wide variety of symptoms and can be misdiagnosed.

Among striking examples of misdiagnosis, there is the experience of one large upstate New York hospital with a group of twenty-three patients. Some came to the hospital seeking help on their own; most were hospitalized on referral from physicians.

Over half had complained of weakness, breathing difficulty, weight loss, and loss of appetite. Some had experienced fatigability, abdominal pain, chest pain, cough, unsteadiness, burning or tingling sensations, dizziness, vomiting, constipation, or sore tongue.

Pallor was common. So were abnormal gait, memory impairment, and other nervous system symptoms.

It was to turn out that all had the same problem, even though not exactly the same symptoms, and in not one case had the right diagnosis been made prior to hospitalization. All twenty-three had pernicious anemia.

Why had the diagnosis been missed by the referring physicians, who in some instances had observed patients over periods of weeks or months? One reason may have been that pernicious anemia has often been considered to be an anemia in which invariably tongue inflammation and abnormal sensations or numbness of the legs are present. But only three of the patients complained of sore tongue and only five had abnormal sensations.

Also, some physicians may be unaware that pernicious anemia is really a multisystem disease. The lack of B_{12} can affect not only the blood but other tissues and systems of the body—liver, digestive system, nervous system, and brain.

Several patients in whom the deficiency aggravated existing anginal chest pain and coronary artery disease were diagnosed as simply having heart disease. Patients with weakness, memory impairment, and difficulty in walking, especially if they were older, were considered to be victims of generalized artery hardening.

Pernicious anemia can be diagnosed readily enough, if suspected, with the aid of laboratory tests.

Blood cell formation may also suffer from lack of another vitamin, folic acid. Folic acid deficiency anemia may develop as the result of disorders that impair absorption of the vitamin from the intestine or from excessive alcohol intake, which interferes with body metabolism, or use, of the vitamin.

Some drugs may lead to the deficiency. One, methotrexate,

which is used for treating cancer and some cases of severe psoriasis, and some drugs used for epilepsy may be responsible.

Not least of all, eating habits may be responsible. Although folic acid is present in many natural foods—leafy vegetables, yeast, liver, eggs, cottage cheese—the vitamin is rapidly destroyed by heat. A deficiency can occur when leafy vegetables, flesh foods, and liver are lacking in the diet or are cooked too long.

Like vitamin B_{12} deficiency, folic acid deficiency is readily diagnosable by blood tests. And administration of the vitamin usually produces prompt response.

Bone marrow depression and reduction in new red cell formation sometimes may be associated with chronic infection such as tuberculosis or sinusitis, or with inflammatory conditions such as rheumatoid arthritis. In addition to supportive measures, including adequate diet and vitamins, treatment should be aimed at combating the infection, inflammation, or other underlying problem.

POLYCYTHEMIA

Polycythemia is a blood disorder quite the reverse of anemia. It involves an excess of red blood cells.

Fatigability, difficulty in concentration, forgetfulness, drowsiness, headache, and vertigo may be among the first symptoms. If uncontrolled, polycythemia may have serious consequences. Life-threatening clots or hemorrhages and little strokes or even a major stroke may develop.

Polycythemia can occur at any age, but the average age of onset is sixty. Men are more often affected than women, and the disease is more common in people of Jewish extraction.

In the disorder, blood-forming tissues in the bone marrow overgrow. And, as an abnormally large number of red cells are produced, the blood thickens and its flow is impeded.

Once suspected, polycythemia can be readily diagnosed by blood tests. And treatment can relieve symptoms and prolong life. Venesection, or blood-letting, is often used and may be needed at first once or twice a week, later at intervals of three or four months. In some cases, in addition to or instead of venesection, injections of radiophosphorus may be used to irradiate the rapidly dividing red cells and bring their numbers under control. Drugs such as busulfan or melphalan may be of value.

Only very recently, evidence has been reported that excessive smoking may be responsible for polycythemia. In many cases it may, in fact, rank as a major cause.

Tobacco smoke has high levels of carbon monoxide. And carbon monoxide has high affinity for hemoglobin; it can actually replace oxygen in hemoglobin. Thus, excessive, sustained exposure to carbon monoxide from smoking can deprive body tissues of adequate supplies of oxygen. In response, the body tries to compensate by producing more red cells, causing polycythemia.

There have been studies in which the hematocrits—the volume percentages of red cells in whole blood—of blood donors who smoked were found to be significantly higher than those of nonsmoking donors.

In 1978, Drs. J. Robert Smith and Stephen A. Landaw of the State University of New York Upstate Medical Center and the Veterans Administration Hospital, Syracuse, reported a study of eighteen men and four women, all with polycythemia, and all excessive cigarette or cigar smokers. Three stopped smoking and two others markedly reduced their smoking. In all five, red blood cell volumes returned to normal and symptoms disappeared within several days. The other patients, still smoking, continued to be polycythemic. "Considering the wide use of tobacco," the physicians noted, "smoking should be one of the largest single causes of polycythemia."

INFLAMMATORY ARTERY DISEASE

Some years ago, physicians at Seattle's Virginia Mason Clinic, a noted diagnostic center, became aware that they were seeing a considerable number of elderly patients who arrived in the same hopeless state of mind and with similar symptoms.

They had crippling muscular pain, weakness, and low-grade fever. They looked and felt depressed. Many had already been to three or four physicians and had spent hundreds of dollars for laboratory work that failed to reveal any cause for their problems.

Two investigators at the clinic, Drs. Kenneth R. Wilske and Louis A. Healey, both also on the faculty of the University of Washington School of Medicine in Seattle, found that for some of the patients the symptoms had started a few months after a bout of flu. Others said they had simply awakened one day with severe muscular pain such as one might expect after a day of unaccustomed hard physical labor—but there had been no such labor.

The two physicians found that the pain usually was in the neck, shoulders, and upper arms, and mild anemia was present; but there was no evidence of rheumatoid arthritis or of malignancy. In every case, however, the blood sedimentation rate was high.

At that point, the investigators wondered if they might be dealing with a syndrome, or set of symptoms, called polymyalgia rheumatica. Although it had come in for little attention in the United States, the condition was well known in Europe, where, according to some estimates, it was as common as gout in the general population and half as common as rheumatoid arthritis in older people.

Aware that a British researcher had suggested that polymyalgia might be identical with early temporal giant cell arteritis—an inflammation of the temporal artery in the head—Wilske and

Healey took biopsies (small tissue samples of the artery for microscopic study). But arteritis was present in only about one-
fourth of the samples.

Nevertheless the two men decided to try the treatment used
for temporal arteritis, which produces as its chief symptoms
headache, and pain and tenderness at the inflamed sites. Within
days after they began injecting a cortisonelike drug, prednisone,
there were dramatic results. One patient, previously confined
to a wheelchair, was up and out of it within three days.

On the average, the patients were back to normal after a month
or two, and most thereafter were maintained on small doses
of prednisone.

Polymyalgia rheumatica and temporal arteritis, the two physicians reported, are two different expressions of giant cell arteritis.

Since the first Mason Clinic report, other studies there and
at other centers have confirmed the effectiveness of prednisone
treatment. They have also indicated that giant cell arteritis can
sometimes be responsible for other problems, including liver
damage, stroke, and personality changes.

One of a series of patients with liver involvement seen at the
Mayo Clinic was a sixty-seven-year-old woman who for a six
month period had been experiencing increasing fatigue, appetite
loss, aching of shoulders and hips, morning stiffness, and pounding headaches. Circulation in several arteries, including the temporal, was impaired, and no pulse at all could be felt in one
arm. Laboratory tests also revealed changes in liver function.
Within a week after prednisone treatment was started she was
free of all symptoms, and within eight weeks her liver function
was back to normal. The prednisone was gradually decreased
in dosage and discontinued after eighteen months.

The various studies indicate that giant cell arteritis mostly
affects people over fifty and usually over sixty-five, women more
commonly than men.

When the temporal artery is affected, symptoms include severe headache, tenderness, and swelling, and commonly there is intermittent jaw pain. A serious complication that may develop if treatment is not instituted is blocking of blood circulation to the optic nerve or retina of the eye, leading to vision loss.

When the disease affects other than the temporal artery, muscular pain is a common symptom. There may be severe aching in neck, back, shoulder, upper arm, hip and thigh muscles. Morning stiffness may be marked. The pain and stiffness are in the muscles, not the joints.

Physical examination reveals nothing specific. Clearly the patient looks ill, uncomfortable, and depressed, but muscles and joints look and feel normal. The clue to diagnosis is a very rapid sedimentation rate.

Because patients complain of appetite loss and lassitude, and because their muscular aches seem diffuse and physical examination shows nothing specific, many patients may be thought to have senile depression or psychosomatic aches and pains. But measurement of the sedimentation rate could help establish the true diagnosis and treatment with a cortisonelike agent such as prednisone can bring relief.

What causes giant cell arteritis is still not clear. But with effective treatment available, Dr. Wilske's admonition is worth heeding by patients and their families and physicians: "When older people begin to fail, giant cell arteritis is one of the first diseases that should be considered, and not one of the last."

7

Turning Down the Pressure

In an unusual decade-long study, investigators at Duke University Center for the Study of Aging and Human Development followed 202 volunteers, all in their sixties and seventies at the start.

At the beginning, and then every two and a half years, they went through two days of careful examinations. Along with many laboratory and other tests, blood pressure measurements were made. Intelligence, too, as indicated by the standard Wechsler Adult Intelligence Scale, was evaluated.

At the end of the ten years, a relationship between blood pressure and maintenance or decline in intelligence was clear. Subjects who had normal pressures showed almost no intellectual decline over the period, while those with elevated pressures had drops of almost ten points in scores.

In pointing up the role of hypertension—high blood pressure—in mental decline, the Duke study added one more important particular to an already serious indictment.

Hypertension is a major health problem, startlingly prevalent. According to latest estimates by the National High Blood Pressure Education Program, the number of Americans with significant blood pressure elevation has reached 35 million.

While hypertension can occur at any age, it has its highest incidence in older people. To age twenty-four, 10.9 percent of men and 1.4 percent of women have elevated pressure. By age fifty-four, 15.3 percent of women and 17.7 percent of men are affected; by age sixty-four, 24.3 percent of women and 27.5 percent of men; and after age seventy-five, 28.3 percent of women and 26.7 percent of men.

Hypertension ranks as our greatest single cause of death and a major cause of disability.

In people with elevated pressure, heart attacks are three to five times more common than in those with normal blood pressure; stroke is four times more common; congestive heart failure is five times more common; and the risk of kidney failure is greatly increased.

Both directly, as the Duke study suggests, and in all of these ways, since disturbances elsewhere in the body can affect the brain, hypertension may take a toll in mental functioning, contributing to the senility problem. But needlessly.

For hypertension is one of the most readily correctable of all body aberrations, but one of the most commonly neglected. Many who have it don't know they do; many who do know are not being treated adequately or at all. Much less than half—only 28 percent—of all hypertensives in the country are being adequately controlled.

The Normal and the High

Blood pressure is simply the force exerted against the walls of arteries as blood flows through. The pressure is produced primarily by the pumping action of the heart and is needed for pushing the body's five quarts of blood through more than 60,000 miles of blood vessels.

The body has a finely tuned system for regulating the pressure and making it responsive to changing demands. When, for example, you lie down, less blood pressure is required because there is less force of gravity to work against, and the pressure automatically is turned down. When you stand up, more pressure is needed—and automatically supplied. Similarly pressure changes occur as needed when you work, play, and eat, and when you are affected by fear, anger, and other emotions.

Many factors are influential in regulating blood pressure. Nervous system stimuli can increase or decrease pressure by constricting or expanding blood vessels. Hormones such as epinephrine and norepinephrine from the adrenal glands atop the kidneys are powerful constrictors of blood vessels and therefore pressure raisers; they are secreted during vigorous physical activity and also during emotional stress. Specialized groups of pressure-sensitive cells, called baroreceptors, scattered through the arterial system, act much like thermostats in homes, except that instead of keeping heat in a preset range they keep pressure within appropriate limits.

But one or more mechanisms for controlling blood pressure may go awry.

How high is high pressure?

Each time the heart beats, pressure increases; and this upper pressure is known as the systolic pressure (systolic, from the Greek for contraction). The pressure at its lowest point, when the heart relaxes between beats, is the diastolic pressure (from the Greek for expansion).

Normal systolic pressure of a person at rest is in the range of 100 to 140, and the normal diastolic is 60 to 90. A blood pressure reading is expressed by both figures, with systolic over diastolic: 140/90, for example.

Because blood pressure varies normally under different circumstances, a single reading above 140/90 does not indicate abnormal pressure. But when the pressure is continuously elevated, a person is considered to have hypertension.

Events and Effects

Hypertension has been called the silent disease for good reason. It is stealthy—easy enough for a physician taking measurements to uncover but not for a victim otherwise to realize that he or she has it.

Mild elevations—and often severe ones—may produce no symptoms at all for long periods. Even when symptoms occur—headaches, dizziness, fatigue, weakness—they may not be recognized as being related to elevated pressure, because they are symptoms common to many other disorders.

But even while not producing symptoms, pressure elevation over a prolonged period can have serious effects.

With pressure elevated, the heart must work harder to pump blood. As a consequence, the heart muscle thickens and increases in size. This is reflected in enlargement of the heart, and the enlargement can be seen on x-ray film. The phenomenon is not strange. Exercise any muscle strenuously—the biceps in your arms, for example—and girth increases.

For a time, despite the increased work burden, the heart accommodates and does well. But there comes a point when it fatigues and is no longer fully able to meet the strain. The result is congestive heart failure (see Chapter 6).

Hypertension may also have another effect on the heart. When a muscle increases in girth, as does the hypertensive heart, the blood vessels supplying it may not increase in size. Those—the coronaries—supplying the heart muscle do not. They have spare capacity, and up to a point that may suffice. But in some cases the burden on the heart is so great that its needs for blood outdistance the spare capacity of the coronaries.

As a result, there may be coronary insufficiency, with chest pain (angina pectoris) or even death of some tissue in an area of heart muscle (myocardial infarction).

The effects of persistent hypertension can extend elsewhere. The kidneys may suffer from reduced blood supply, which impairs their ability to function at full capacity. They become less effective in ridding the body of waste products and have an increased tendency to retain instead of properly excrete salt. Salt tends to attract water, so there is abnormal fluid retention, which increases the chances for heart failure.

Kidney damage from elevated pressure may also include gradual destruction of the tiny filtration units within the kidneys where urine is formed. As more and more are destroyed, kidney function deteriorates seriously, and eventually the kidneys may fail completely, causing uremic poisoning and death.

Hypertention also has serious effects on arteries.

Put any pumping system under strain and you are likely to increase the rate of wear not only on the pump but also on the pipelines. If, say, a system is designed to take a maximum strain of a hundred pounds, it will last longer if the strain never does get that high. If the strain persistently exceeds one hundred pounds, the system will deteriorate.

One form of deterioration in the blood pipelines, the arteries, is rupture or blowout. After long periods of excessive pressure, an area of artery wall may become so weakened that it finally blows out. This is most likely to occur in brain arteries, which are not so well embedded in firm, protective surrounding tissues as are many other arteries elsewhere in the body.

A brain hemorrhage, resulting from rupture of an artery within the brain, is one form of cerebrovascular accident, or stroke.

In addition to hemorrhaging within the brain and the resulting destruction of brain substance and stroke, an accident may occur outside the brain (subarachnoid hemorrhage) when small outpouchings of artery wall at the base of the brain rupture and cause massive bleeding and death.

Another complication of very high pressure can be hypertensive encephalopathy, in which the brain substance swells, causing violent headaches, disturbances of brain function, and sometimes coma.

Brain arteries are also subject to another problem, just as are the coronary arteries of the heart and other major arteries in the body: atherosclerosis, the clogging of arteries by deposits on inner walls.

When clogging of brain arteries progresses, it may produce

little strokes as circulation is reduced; and when the clogging reaches the point of cutting off blood supply to a brain area, a massive stroke results. Brain tissue dies just as does heart muscle tissue when atherosclerosis finally cuts off circulation to part of the heart muscle.

And high blood pressure has come to be recognized recently as an important factor in atherosclerosis.

The Role in Artery Disease

Perhaps no other health question has produced as much thoughtful controversy within the medical profession and so much confusion in the public mind as what provokes the accumulation of clogging deposits on artery walls.

Once, atherosclerosis was considered to be something that just happened with aging—an inevitability. But then came such discoveries as these: That, at any age, the Bantu people in South Africa are remarkably free of atherosclerosis; so it could hardly be inevitable. And that young American soldiers killed in the Korean War, many still in their teens, showed significant atherosclerosis upon autopsy. So age was not a critical factor.

At various times, many different factors have been espoused as *the* cause. But it is now recognized that the artery disease is not a result of any one factor but rather of varied factors that may interact.

Modern diet, of course, containing high levels of cholesterol and fats, has been blamed for years. Cholesterol is found in atherosclerotic deposits. The waxy material, a natural—and important—body substance produced by the liver, has many roles, including regulating the passage of materials into and out of body cells and as an ingredient required for the production of essential hormones. Up to a point, then, cholesterol is vital; but too much can cause trouble.

It's now well known that some of our most commonly used

foods—meat and dairy products, which are high in saturated fats; and eggs and organ meats, which are high in cholesterol— can, if used to excess, raise the level of cholesterol in the blood.

Obesity is another factor. With excess weight, there is increased likelihood of elevated blood cholesterol. In fact, one recent study suggests that total calories may be more important than fats or cholesterol in the diet in elevating blood fat levels.

In the study of 4057 adults in Tecumseh, Michigan, made by Drs. Allen B. Nichols and Leon D. Ostrander of the University of Michigan School of Medicine, tallies were made of the consumption of 110 different food items; of average consumption of foods high in fat, starch, sugar, and alcohol; and of total daily caloric intake.

It turned out that cholesterol and fat levels in the blood did not particularly correlate with the kind of diet—but did with total calories and body fat. Excessive caloric intake—too much eating—leading to weight gain and body fat accumulation is more important, the study found, in raising blood fat levels than the proportions of fat, starch, sugar, or alcohol in the diet.

Cigarette smoking has been indicated, as the result of autopsy studies, as causing a significant increase in the degree of atherosclerosis.

Modern sedentary living appears to be a factor. Many studies have indicated that men who get regular exercise run a lesser risk of heart attack than those who do not. Exercise is an aid in avoiding overweight and in taking off weight. Evidence has also been found that exercise may help reduce blood fat levels.

But, increasingly, investigators have been assigning a critical role to high blood pressure in fostering atherosclerosis.

One clue to the importance of hypertension lies in the pulmonary artery phenomenon. Running from heart to lungs, a short distance, the pulmonary arteries end in a great network of capillaries, the tiniest of blood vessels, in the lungs. It is through the thin capillary walls that oxygen and carbon dioxide diffuse, and a great network is needed since the purpose of the lungs is to exchange oxygen for carbon dioxide. Because the capillaries can accommodate large amounts of blood, they offer little resistance to blood flow.

And so blood pressure in the pulmonary arteries does not need to be nearly as high as elsewhere—and in fact is as low as 35/15.

And the pulmonary arteries have another notable distinction. Almost never does atherosclerosis occur in them no matter how much may be present elsewhere in the body. Yet the pulmonary arteries are subject to the same influences as the other arteries— diet, obesity, smoking. All, that is, except one: hypertension.

Exactly how hypertension promotes atherosclerosis is still not clear. One possible way is by the abnormal pounding that elevated pressure exerts on the arterial inner linings, sufficient, some investigators believe, to disrupt the lining surfaces, opening the way for deposits to be laid down.

But in any case the association between hypertension and atherosclerosis seems clear. Many studies have shown that a very large proportion of people who experience heart attacks—an end result of atherosclerosis of the coronary arteries of the heart—have elevated pressure. In the government's long-term study in Framingham, Massachusetts, men and women with normal pressure experienced only one-fourth the rate of coronary heart disease generally found among people of their age and sex.

At the University of Pittsburgh, Dr. Campbell Moses looked for atherosclerotic deposits during some 500 autopsies and found a much greater incidence and degree of severity in the coronary and brain arteries of people who had been hypertensive.

In some animal experiments, drugs have been used to induce hypertension. Investigators then have tied off a carotid artery on one side of the neck while the carotid on the other side was left intact and continued to supply blood to that side of the brain. Atherosclerosis was found to develop on the untied-off side as a result of the high pressure transmitted to brain vessels, but it did not develop on the tied-off side.

Controlling the Pressure

In only about 10 percent of all cases of hypertension can some specific underlying organic problem be found. It can be a faulty kidney artery, a constriction or narrowing of the aorta, the body's main trunkline artery, or a benign tumor of an adrenal gland atop a kidney. In such cases, it is often possible for surgical correction of the abnormality to end the hypertension once and for all.

Even though a curable cause cannot be found in 90 percent of hypertensives, almost invariably hypertension can be controlled effectively.

In some cases, loss of excess weight by itself—or sometimes coupled with a reduction of salt intake—is enough to normalize the pressure.

In others, drug treatment works if given a chance. Many antihypertensive drugs are available. Diuretic drugs act to lower pressure by increasing the kidneys' excretion of sodium and reducing fluid retention, thus reducing blood volume toward normal levels. Other drugs act to reduce the flow of exciting impulses that cause blood vessel constriction and elevation of pressure.

The value of drug treatment has been shown by many studies.

One of the most important was the Veterans Administration Study Group's trials in seventeen VA hospitals with 523 men with an average age of fifty-one years. Of the 523, 143 had substantial pressure elevations, with diastolic pressures of 115 to 129. The remaining 380 had only relatively mild elevations, with diastolic pressures of 90 through 114.

The men were divided, some receiving antihypertensive medication, while the remainder, for comparison, received placebos (look-alike but inert preparations).

In the higher pressure group, with pressures of 115 to 129, the difference in outcome between treated and controls was so great and the incidence of morbid events in the control or comparison group was so high that the investigators judged it necessary on ethical grounds to stop the study prematurely and place the placebo group on medication.

During the course of the trial, twenty-seven severe complicating events occurred in the patients on placebos as compared to two in the treated men. The events included heart attacks, major and minor strokes, and heart failure. Four deaths occurred in the placebo group, none in the treated.

Nor could there have been a much more impressive demonstration of the value of treating mild hypertension than in the results in the 380 men with pressures of 90 to 114. Compared with the men who did not receive treatment but served as controls, those put on drug treatment showed a two-thirds reduction in the risk of developing stroke or heart attack; and where a sizable proportion of the untreated patients went on to progress from mild to severe hypertension, none of the treated patients did.

But there have been problems standing in the way of effective treatment for all who need it.

The problems. For one thing, many who have hypertension, as mentioned earlier, do not know they have it, and will not know until the pressure is measured—a simple, painless measurement done in a few minutes.

For another, the best treatment requires custom tailoring to the individual patient. The right medication in the right dosage has to be found to bring down the pressure with minimal or no side effects.

As with any other drugs, antihypertensive agents can cause unpleasant effects in patients who happen to be particularly sensitive to them. The side effects differ with different drugs. Among them are depressed feelings, headaches, lethargy, weakness, mouth dryness, faintness, nausea, and impotence.

Yet the right drug—or combination of drugs—in the right dosage usually can be found, sometimes luckily in the beginning, sometimes after some experimentation.

Unfortunately, many people experiencing a side effect at the beginning of treatment stop right there. Unless they realize very clearly that although they may be experiencing no symptoms from the elevated pressure, they will eventually feel the consequences, they are quick to stop treatment when it makes them feel worse than they felt before—even though with further trial a more suitable treatment could be found.

And even when suitable treatment is found, taking medication regularly, with the prospect of having to take it for a lifetime, can seem like more of a chore than a benediction unless the full importance of controlling hypertension is understood.

And that importance for older people includes not only minimizing the risk of death or disability from stroke, kidney failure, and heart disease, but also minimizing the risk of intellectual decline.

Yet there are other problems when it comes to the control of hypertension in older people: several still-prevalent myths.

The myths. One of these is that older people tolerate their high blood pressure well; for them, it is of little consequence.

That is not true. In addition to the Duke study, which has shown the relationship between blood pressure elevation and mental decline in people in their sixties and seventies, the Framingham study has clearly shown the significance of blood pressure levels for health and survival in the elderly.

And the Framingham study has laid to rest—or should have if attention was paid to its results—other myths and misconceptions.

The Framingham study is a unique long-term investigation. Formally known as the Heart Disease Epidemiology Study, it was begun in 1949 by the National Heart Institute in the town of Framingham, Massachusetts, and has been following closely what happens to more than 5000 men and women in that community. A major objective has been to determine which of them (all healthy at the start) would develop evidence of coronary heart disease and to try to establish what factors led to the disease.

The 2292 men and 2845 women who took part were aged thirty through fifty-nine at the start. And for each of them detailed observations were made to determine life habits, environmental characteristics, familial traits, and other factors that might conceivably turn out to be related in any way to the development of cardiovascular disease. Every two years, the subjects went through a thorough ninety-minute physical examination that included electrocardiographic studies and blood pressure measurements.

Over the years, some of the people have remained remarkably healthy; others have had heart attacks and strokes. And keeping track, investigators found that overweight is a factor related to anginal chest pain and sudden death. They found that smoking increases the risk of heart attack and sudden death. They found that elevated levels of blood fats are associated with increased risk. They found that decreased physical activity—sedentary living—increases the heart disease risk.

And they found that elevated blood pressure stood out as a prime risk-increasing factor.

Heart attacks proved to be three to five times more common in Framingham people with hypertension than in others. The risk of coronary heart disease and its manifestations—including angina, heart attack, and sudden death—was impressively related to the blood pressure level.

And the risk of stroke proved to be four times as high among those who had hypertension, even though they had no symptoms of hypertension, as among those with normal pressure.

And what of the importance of hypertension in the elderly? The Framingham data show that even in old age, in both men and women, hypertension is the most significant of controllable risk factors. Even small elevations increase the incidence of coronary heart disease and stroke. The Framingham data show that the *elderly tolerate high pressures less well, not better, than younger people.*

Two other long-accepted notions have been shown to be myths by the Framingham study data. One is that blood pressure normally rises with age. The fact: in many people, blood pressure does not change with age.

The other misconception: that only the diastolic pressure is important.

The assumption about diastolic pressure's importance has been based on the idea that while the systolic pressure is the higher pressure, occurring with the heartbeat at the moment when blood is ejected from the heart into the arteries, the diastolic, or between-beat, pressure is still the one to which the arteries are subjected for the longest periods. So it seemed that the diastolic, if elevated, might produce the major share of damage.

Also, it had long been believed that systolic pressure in particular tends to go up with age—so much so that the common belief has been that when systolic pressure equals the sum of 100 and a person's age, it is normal systolic pressure.

But a sixty-year-old with 160 systolic or a seventy-year-old with 170 no longer can be considered to have normal pressure.

Systolic pressure does not necessarily increase *normally* with age, and the Framingham data prove it to be as important as the diastolic. They show that at any diastolic pressure—low, normal, or high—risk of coronary disease or stroke rises as systolic pressure increases.

And, contrary to conventional belief, the effects of high blood pressure are the same in elderly women as in older men. Women are *not* more tolerant of hypertension. And this is true in terms of systolic pressure. Women with normal diastolic but only borderline or somewhat elevated systolic pressures have a risk of heart disease 50 percent above standard. At any level of pressure, men and women have about the same risk of stroke.

Dr. Adrian M. Ostfeld and his colleagues at Yale University

School of Medicine studied high blood pressure and risk of stroke in 3400 people aged sixty-five to seventy-four. One half were men and one half women. The investigators found that the risk of stroke rose with increasing levels of both systolic and diastolic pressure. And those whose diastolic pressure was normal showed a tripling of stroke incidence as systolic pressures rose from less than 139 to 160 or greater.

Do older people respond as well to treatment for high blood pressure as younger people? They clearly do.

We mentioned the VA Study Group trials earlier. In addition to showing the benefit of treatment at all ages, they show the benefit in patients over sixty.

In the group with only slightly elevated pressures, there were ten strokes in those over sixty receiving placebos, three in those receiving treatment. In the placebo group, ten patients developed congestive heart failure; no treated patient did.

Among those over sixty who had greater elevations of pressure, there were ten morbid events—strokes and heart problems—and one death in the placebo group; there were no morbid events and no deaths in the treated patients.

In a recent special report on the elderly hypertensive patient appearing in the *New York State Journal of Medicine,* Dr. Ostfeld of Yale noted that we are repeatedly told about the many millions of Americans with high blood pressure, "But we consistently neglect the fact that 40 percent of these hypertensive cases are past age 60.

"Not only hypertension but all of its consequences are concentrated in the elderly. The great majority of strokes, heart attacks, and episodes of congestive heart failure occur in those over 60, and the death rates in these disorders are highest in the same age group.

"The present relative unconcern about hypertension in the elderly could be more easily justified if there were nothing we could do about it. It is true that most of the classic risk factors, such as diet, smoking, and blood lipids, have little effect on disease incidence past age 60. But the effect of hypertension as a risk factor is stronger than at an earlier age. And it is clear that high blood pressure can be controlled in the elderly with resultant decline in morbidity and mortality rates."

8

Solving the
Gland Problems

They made up a group of patients coming under special study by University of North Carolina Medical School investigators.

Fatigue, irritability, anxiety, and depression were common complaints. Some had been experiencing impairment of recent memory and difficulties in concentrating. A few suffered from delusions of being persecuted.

In their performances on a series of tests, they appeared to be "strongly similar" to patients with proven organic brain changes.

But they were given other tests, and those for thyroid gland function disclosed hyperthyroidism, a disorder of excessive gland functioning and thyroid hormone production. Striking improvement in all their symptoms followed treatment for hyperthyroidism.

That brain as well as body functioning is influenced by hormone secretions of the thyroid—and of other endocrine glands—has long been known.

Yet the responsibility of malfunctioning glands for symptoms mimicking those of organic dementia is not always recognized—a potentially tragic failure because the malfunctioning is very often correctable.

THE THYROID

According to an old medical saying—and it exaggerates only a little—just a few grams of thyroid hormone can make the difference between an Einstein and an idiot.

Thyroid hormone secretions total less than a spoonful in a year. Yet they control body metabolism—the rate at which chemical processes go on and energy is used. They are needed for normal functioning of the heart and circulatory system and for the health of muscles and sensitivity of nerves.

Their critical role in brain development used to be obvious in cretinism, a congenital absence of thyroid secretions. A cretin baby failed to thrive, exhibited torpid behavior and, within a year or two, mental retardation. Today, with tests to recognize cretinism early, the once-inevitable consequences can be avoided by thyroid hormone treatment.

Total lack of thyroid hormone is rare. But thyroid malfunctioning—production of either too much or too little secretion—is relatively common.

Especially when the malfunctioning is extreme, manifestations may be unmistakable.

With severe hyperthyroidism—excessive thyroid secretion—the victim may be nervous and irritable and tire easily. Emaciation may develop despite a good appetite. Often the eyes protrude, the skin is warm and moist, the pulse may race, and blood pressure may shoot up.

In the other direction, the severely hypothyroid person—whose gland produces grossly inadequate secretions—may experience weakness, listlessness, and memory impairment. In addition, speech may become slow and thick, the skin dry, and unusual sensitivity to cold temperature may occur.

Usually, such classic symptoms of severe thyroid malfunctioning are quickly recognized for what they are by physicians and sometimes by patients themselves. Blood and other tests of thyroid function can confirm the diagnosis, and treatment can be gratifyingly effective.

For hyperthyroidism, a drug such as propylthiouracil or methimazole may be used. Over a period of months, the drug suppresses excessive secretion, bringing thyroid function down to a normal range, at which point treatment can be stopped. Alternatively, in some cases, surgery or radioactive iodine treatment may be preferable. Surgery—subtotal thyroidectomy—removes part of the gland, enough to eliminate excess secretion. Injection of radioactive iodine may also bring thyroid activity down to normal.

For hypothyroidism, simple replacement therapy with thyroid pills effectively supplements inadequate gland production.

But thyroid problems are not always quickly or readily recognized. They do not always take classic forms.

Hyperthyroidism

One example of how misleading hyperthyroidism sometimes can be in an older person is a woman who was finally hospitalized after a year of losing weight and suffering from weakness and episodes of diarrhea. By the time she was admitted, she weighed only sixty-five pounds.

At first she was thought to have a gastrointestinal cancer, but tests ruled that out. Still she went right on losing weight in the hospital, remaining a diagnostic puzzle until finally, two weeks after admission, the possibility of thyroid disease was considered and quickly confirmed by tests. The diagnosis had been overlooked at first because she had no classic indications of hyperthyroidism—no gland enlargement or sweating, for example. After thyroid treatment, she rapidly regained weight and strength.

In another case in the same hospital, an elderly man soon

after admission was sent off to the psychiatric ward for evaluation of what appeared to be a serious mental disturbance. For a year he had become increasingly unmanageable at home, subject to episodes of agitation, restlessness, and overactivity. Sometimes he became combative; occasionally he had delusions.

In the psychiatric ward, his restlessness continued. He could not sit still, insisted upon mopping floors, washing windows, busing trays, and he rarely slept. After several weeks of this, one physician on the ward finally suspected the possibility of thyroid disorder and ordered tests, which clearly showed severe hyperthyroidism, which responded to treatment.

Investigators studying hyperthyroid patients have reported that in as many as 20 percent there is serious mental disturbance—but not uniform in type.

In one University of North Carolina study of a series of ten patients with mental disturbances related to hyperthyroidism, four had increased difficulty in concentration and impairment of recent memory. Many had difficulty doing simple arithmetic. Fatigue, anxiety, and irritability were common. Two patients suffered from depression and two from delusions of persecution. In all of them, treatment for the thyroid problem led to recovery.

Hyperthyroidism can occur at any time of life. But a growing mass of new data, as Dr. Paul J. Davis of the State University of New York School of Medicine at Buffalo has recently reported, suggests that as many as one-third of all hyperthyroid patients are older than sixty years.

And, especially in older patients, detection of the gland disorder can demand alertness.

In contrast to younger hyperthyroid patients, as many as one-third of elderly patients may have no goiter or obvious gland enlargement. Some even have an apathetic appearance that disguises the problem. And laboratory findings in the elderly sometimes can be confounding, with one test suggesting that the thyroid is normal, a mistake only to be discovered when other laboratory tests indicate abnormality.

Hypothyroidism

Underfunctioning of the thyroid gland can occur at any age, but it is primarily a disorder of the fifth, sixth, and seventh decades of life.

Yet its recognition in older people is often handicapped because it is insidious in onset; and for a long time its victims—and sometimes their physicians—may fail to appreciate that a process is going on that is distinct from "growing older."

A state of low thyroid functioning was identified only about a century ago in England and was originally called myxedema. And in 1883, a special British medical commission was appointed to look into the strange condition.

Five years later, after studying a hundred cases, the committee issued a report in which it noted that all the myxedematous patients were slow in thought and response, suffered from poor memory, and some had delusions, hallucinations, or frank insanity.

More than a dozen years later, Dr. G. R. Murray, a British physician who was the first to treat myxedema successfully, published his *A System of Medicine* in which he detailed how the symptoms developed.

Often first to appear, he noted, was listlessness, so that ordinary routine daily activities previously performed without any great effort took more and more effort and became irksome. Commonly, sensitivity to cold followed. Later, in virtually all cases came a growing slowness in being able to comprehend a new subject or follow a new line of thought. Irritability, too, was common. And unless treatment was started early, Murray pointed out, mania, melancholia, or dementia might develop.

When hypothyroidism is extreme, it can produce physical changes which, taken together, point almost unmistakably to what is wrong.

Along with progressive slowing of mental and physical activities, there may be an increase in weight, decrease in appetite, a masklike facial appearance, thickening and rigidity of the skin, which also may become dry, cold, rough, and scaly. The upper eyelids may become waterlogged and the eyebrows elevated in efforts to keep the eyes open. The hair may become coarse, brittle, and may tend to fall out.

But such a concatenation of symptoms may not be present in mild to moderate hypothyroidism and even inevitably in advanced cases.

And older patients and their families—and sometimes their physicians—may be fooled into believing that any physical symptoms may be a normal part of growing older and that mental symptoms may reflect senile brain changes.

At the University of North Carolina, where investigators looked into mental changes accompanying hyperthyroidism, they also studied a series of patients with mental changes accompanying hypothyroidism.

One elderly woman with low thyroid functioning suffered from confusion and depression, another from confusion and great anxiety. Most of the patients complained of poor recent memory and difficulty in concentrating. Several women complained they no longer could remember cooking recipes they had used most of their adult lives. Some had difficulty remembering where they placed things around the house.

With thyroid treatment, such symptoms quickly disappeared.

At any time of life—and particularly in the later years—the possibility that thyroid disturbance may be responsible for mental as well as physical problems, with the mental sometimes overshadowing the physical, deserves consideration.

Parathyroid Disturbances

These, too, can contribute to what may seem to be mental problems associated with senility as well as to varied physical symptoms.

The parathyroid glands are four small bodies attached to the thyroid gland in the neck area. They secrete parathormone, a hormone important in regulating the balance of calcium in the body.

Calcium is the most abundant mineral in the body. It comes from milk and other foods. It goes into the formation of bones and teeth. A constant level is needed in the blood in order to maintain normal heartbeat, normal clotting time of blood, and normal functioning of muscles and nerves.

When the parathyroid glands function excessively and overse-crete parathyroid hormone, as they do in hyperparathyroidism, levels of calcium in the blood are greatly increased, with the mineral sometimes even being leached out of bones by the excessive hormone activity.

The calcium excess—hypercalcemia—can produce varied symptoms. There may be weakness, appetite loss, nausea, consti-pation, abdominal pain, thirst, and excessive urination. Calcium stones may form in the kidneys.

Hypercalcemia also can produce mental symptoms, including confusion, delusions, retardation, memory impairment, halluci-nations, and sometimes spells of unconsciousness. Even when the hypercalcemia is less severe, it may sometimes be responsible for lassitude; lack of initiative, interest, and spontaneity; and mental depression.

Hyperparathyroidism tends to be more common in older than younger people. Nearly one-third of patients with the problem are older than sixty. It results from either a benign tumor, which often is confined to a single gland, or to simple overgrowth of parathyroid tissue.

Until recently, before development of relatively simple tests for measuring not only calcium but also the amount of parathor-mone in the blood, diagnosis was sometimes difficult. Now, if only the problem is suspected, its diagnosis is a straightforward matter.

Effective treatment is the surgical removal of a parathyroid tumor when that is present or the removal of some of the excess

parathyroid tissue when overgrowth is the cause of excess secretions.

The reverse condition of hypoparathyroidism—with its failure
of the glands to produce adequate amounts of parathyroid hormone and resulting low blood calcium levels—can also produce
physical and mental symptoms.

Hypoparathyroidism may result from accidental removal of
or damage to the parathyroid glands during thyroid gland surgery, and in such cases becomes obvious within twenty-four
hours. There is also a form, called idiopathic hypoparathyroidism, in which the glands are wasted or absent. And there is
still another form, pseudohypoparathyroidism, in which there
is no real deficiency in parathormone but the hormone no longer
is normally effective.

When hypoparathyroidism leads to extremely low calcium
levels in the blood, the result can be tetany, with muscle
spasms which may occur in any muscle but are especially likely
to affect muscles of fingers, toes, face, eyes, tongue, and voice
box.

In idiopathic hypoparathyroidism, about one-third of patients
are intellectually impaired and another third have emotional disturbances, including emotional lability, anxiety, depression, and
irritability.

Treatment is effective. It involves an increased intake of calcium, using a supplement such as calcium gluconate or calcium
carbonate. It also calls for suitable doses of vitamin D, which
has actions somewhat similar to those of parathormone and helps
to raise blood calcium to normal levels.

ADRENAL DISORDERS

When the adrenal glands atop the kidneys become underac-
tive, as they do in Addison's disease, or overactive, as they do
in Cushing's syndrome, many disturbances can ensue—emo-

tional and behavioral as well as physical, with the former some-times the first to become manifest.

The glands play many vital roles through the numerous hor-mones they produce. Some of these hormones influence heart rate, motility in the gastrointestinal tract, and dilation of the pupils of the eyes. Others help control the handling of protein, fat, and carbohydrates; and still others influence the handling of sodium and potassium.

Addison's Disease

This insidious progressive disease, with its hormone insuffi-ciency, occurs in all age groups, including the elderly, and affects both sexes equally.

It may develop when, for unknown reasons, part of the adrenal gland shrivels. In some cases it results from partial gland destruc-tion by inflammation, tuberculosis or other infectious disease, or a malignancy.

Weakness and fatigue are among the early symptoms. Loss of weight and appetite, nausea, vomiting, and diarrhea often occur; sometimes too, episodes of dizziness and fainting. And there may be such symptoms as apathy, lack of interest and initiative, poverty of thought, general negativism, and mental depression.

There is often an increase of skin pigmentation, and there may be black freckles over the face, forehead, neck, and shoul-ders, and bluish black discolorations of lips, mouth, and rectum.

Often Addison's disease is first suspected when increased skin pigmentation is found, but in some cases the increase may be minimal.

There are various tests that can point to Addison's disease. They include blood tests revealing a low white blood cell count, increased levels of blood elements called eosinophiles, and low levels of sodium and high levels of potassium.

In another test, ACTH, a pituitary gland hormone that usually stimulates the adrenal glands, is infused into a vein. If the levels of adrenal hormones in the blood do not rise, that fact points to Addison's.

Addison's disease can be treated effectively with hormones to compensate for the adrenal deficiency, so effectively that even a patient with relatively severe disease can expect to lead a full life.

Cushing's Syndrome

This condition, with its excessive adrenal activity, may result from abnormal growth of part of the glands or from a benign or malignant adrenal tumor. Sometimes, the adrenals pour out too many hormones because they are overstimulated by secretions from a pituitary gland or ovarian tumor.

Here again many symptoms are possible. There may be a "moonlike" fullness of the face, and fat accumulations may appear on the trunk and back. The skin may be thin and quick to bruise. General weakness, distention of the abdomen, unusual growth of body hair, and impairment of sexual function may develop.

And mental disturbances are common. Mental depression is one of the most frequent. But any or several of many others are possible: concentration difficulties, memory impairment, irritability, apathy, excitement, anxiety, disorientation, paranoid delusions.

For diagnosis, measurement of hormone levels in blood and urine is often helpful. Infusing the pituitary hormone ACTH can help in some cases to establish the cause, since an adrenal tumor will not respond to ACTH. Skull x rays can reveal a pituitary tumor. And still other tests are available.

Treatment will depend upon cause. In some cases, irradiation of the pituitary gland is effective. In others, adrenal gland surgery may be needed.

Recently, there have been reports of promising early results in treating Cushing's syndrome with a drug, cyproheptadine. Long used as an antihistamine for hay fever and other allergies, the drug turns out to have other actions as well. It has eliminated symptoms in about 60 percent of Cushing's patients for whom it has been tried.

Pheochromocytoma

This is a tumor, usually benign, of an adrenal gland which can secrete large amounts of adrenal hormones and produce many disturbances. It has its greatest incidence between the third and fifth decades but can occur at any age.

Almost always, a pheochromocytoma produces high blood pressure, which may be persistent or may come and go in abrupt episodes. Severe headache, flushing, cold and clammy skin, chest pain, palpitation, nausea, vomiting, visual disturbances, breathing difficulty, and constipation are among other possible symptoms.

Commonly, pheochromocytoma brings with it a feeling of apprehension and a sense of doom. And in some cases, the first manifestation may be anxiety.

Blood and urine tests are helpful in diagnosis. Surgical removal of the tumor is the treatment. It can usually be delayed with medication until the patient is in optimum physical condition.

9

Detecting and Eliminating the Depressive Influence

She was seventy-eight years old when she was finally hospital-ized—and even then, not because of what had been going on for some time, but because of recent weight loss, abdominal pain, and flatulence. Because the symptoms could have indicated a serious problem, possibly cancer, she was thoroughly studied. But the tests revealed nothing to explain her symptoms.

Nurses, however, did notice that the patient not only ate poorly but showed virtually no interest in her surroundings and what was going on around her.

When her family was questioned on that point, they reported that the symptoms for which she had been hospitalized had come after a period of decline, of gradual loss of interest in everything. She had arrived at the point of no longer wishing to see people. She just sat, silent, immobile, had to be told when to eat and when to go to bed, and often gave no indication of hearing when spoken to. She was, her family thought, "just getting old," suffering from artery hardening.

But with these clues to go on, it wasn't long before physicians in the hospital arrived at a diagnosis: depression, not senile dete-rioration. And when she received treatment for the depression, she was relieved of her physical symptoms and became mentally alert and alive again.

Depression is a problem of staggering proportions. It is responsible, at any age, not only for a vast amount of mental suffering but for much physical suffering as well. Commonly, it can trigger a wide variety of physical illnesses.

It can do that in the young; it can do it in the old. And in the old it can make any symptoms of senility from other causes worse, and it can, not uncommonly, produce senilitylike symptoms when there are no other causes.

Depression, moreover, is no rare problem. It is common at all ages. And it is especially common in older people.

An additional needlessly unhappy fact: It is not unusually difficult to diagnose, yet very commonly it goes undiagnosed for long periods in all age groups; and it is especially likely to go long undiagnosed—and even never diagnosed at all—in older people.

It deserves very careful consideration.

The 8 Million

Almost everyone is familiar with the feeling that comes occasionally of being "down," "blue," "depressed." At such times, nothing seems satisfying, all looks bleak, it is difficult to get oneself to do anything.

Such everyday blues are brief and disappear spontaneously. Their possible causes are many: the weather, a letdown after a holiday, insufficient sleep, excessive work demands and inadequate time to meet them.

Depression, too, quite normally follows loss or separation from a familiar person or place and brings with it feelings of helplessness and hopelessness; but such depression normally subsides spontaneously in a relatively short time.

But depression can be more serious and is for millions. A National Institute of Mental Health survey indicates that as many as 8 million Americans a year suffer depression severe enough to merit treatment.

For depression can produce an incredible range of physical and mental symptoms. There may be overwhelming fatigue, sleeping problems, headaches, loss of appetite, digestive disturbances. The depressed may develop urinary frequency or urgency, heart palpitations, chest constriction, pain in the area of the heart that may seem like an indication of heart trouble. Some experience visual disturbances, ear noises, mouth dryness, numbness and tingling sensations.

In serious depression, there is a chronic change of mood, an extended lowering of spirits, a tired, dull, empty, sad feeling, with loss of enjoyment of relationships and activities that under normal circumstances make life worth living.

And there may be other changes: irritability, indecision, impatience over trivial matters, impaired memory, inability to concentrate, feelings of remorse and guilt.

No one person has all of the symptoms. Some may have a few symptoms very intensely; others a variety less intensely.

Many celebrated people have suffered from depression. Abraham Lincoln went through recurring depressions beginning in young manhood. Nathaniel Hawthorne at one point became so depressed that for twelve years he rarely left his room. He wrote Longfellow, "I have secluded myself from society; and yet I never meant any such thing. I have made a captive of myself and put me into a dungeon, and now I cannot find the key to let myself out."

Winston Churchill called his depressions "my black dog." Once, he recalled, "for two or three years, the light faded out of the picture. . . . I sat in the House of Commons but black depression settled on me."

Much of their suffering could have been relieved today.

Prevalence in Older People

Common at any age, depression may be even more so among the elderly.

A recent review of experiences with patients at Duke University Hospital found that in more than half of all admissions of older patients, depression was the major disorder.

A study some years ago by Dr. E. W. Busse and his associates at Duke found that elderly subjects were aware of more frequent and more annoying depressive periods than they had experienced earlier in life. They reported that during such episodes they felt so discouraged, worried, and troubled that often they saw no reason to continue their existence. Only a small number admitted entertaining suicidal ideas, but a larger percentage did indicate that during such depressive periods they would welcome a painless death.

Since 1955, the Duke Longitudinal Study of Aging has been checking a panel of several hundred men and women, sixty years of age and over at the start, all well adjusted to begin with. Periodically, every two years at first and then later every year, the panel, all volunteers, was examined.

The study found depression to be exceedingly common in these otherwise well-functioning elderly people. At any one time, 20 to 25 percent of them were diagnosed as depressed. After seven to eight periods of evaluation, only 30 percent had no depressive episode, 40 percent had at least one episode, and 30 percent had two or more episodes.

Old age has been called a "season of loss." And depressive reactions are responses to losses. Losses among older people may include declines in physical vigor, mental agility, income, and losses of loved ones.

The Lag in Diagnosis

Even in younger people, depression may long escape diagnosis. Elapsed time from onset of symptoms to accurate recognition of depression has been found in several studies to range from three to thirty-six months, during which the victims, if they receive any treatment at all, are treated for other illnesses, while their difficulties worsen and financial resources are depleted.

At any age, there may be delay in diagnosis because in many cases victims of depression, although aware of their depressed feelings, are much more aware of their physical symptoms. They may attach little importance to their depression of mood, even considering that it is the result rather than cause of physical symptoms. When they seek medical help, they report only the physical symptoms not the mental.

According to some expert estimates, only one in ten persons suffering from depression who could benefit from treatment actually receives it. And among the reasons given by the experts are that many people don't realize that depression is treatable, others don't recognize or acknowledge that they are depressed, and still others consider themselves too worthless to warrant treatment.

And it has been said that self-defeating behavior seems to be built right into the fiber of depression; the unfavorable evaluation of oneself that is characteristic of depression often prevents treatment. Many of the depressed feel that they don't deserve the time, effort, and money required for treatment. Often they feel so depressed that they feel the treatment won't work in their case even if it cures everyone else.

In the elderly, depression may be even more likely to escape prompt detection and treatment—or even detection and treatment at all—for the foregoing reasons and still others.

In the elderly, the symptoms of depression may be thought—by family, friends, victims, and even by some physicians—to be those of hopeless, untreatable senile dementia.

In a fair, reasoned analysis of the problem which appeared recently in the professional journal *Hospital Practice,* Dr. Joy R. Joffe of Johns Hopkins University wrote:

"The physician frequently has to work against a tide of lay misconceptions that contribute to functional disorders. I recall the reaction of a son to my recommendation that his 80-year-old mother be hospitalized so that the proper chemotherapy for depression could be carried out. He resisted.

"I asked: "If your mother were 40, would you question hospitalization? What is so different about being 80? Isn't her time important to her?" He relented, coming to understand that the persisting depression was destructive not only to his mother but to his family with whom she lived.

"Subject to the same kinds of functional disorders as the young, the elderly, regrettably, tend to be abandoned to a degree not only by society but by specialties, such as my own, psychiatry. Some physicians tend to interpret many reversible and treatable functional disorders as irreversible dementia, thus denying the elderly the right to treatment. . . .

"Yet if we look at the facts, we see that the prognosis is excellent for elderly patients with depression or another functional disorder. Such depressions are treatable in various ways, provided someone recognizes the problem and is familiar with the modalities."

And, finally, there appears to be an increasing realization among physicians of the significance and treatability of depression in the elderly—a realization which needs to be communicated clearly to older victims and their families.

"In geriatrics, clinicians are rapidly learning," observes Dr. Leonard Cammer, an authority on depression and clinical associate professor of psychiatry at New York Medical College, "that the weariness with life, irritability, withdrawal, forgetfulness and sleep difficulties in older persons are the symptoms of depression and not the products of 'senility,' 'chronic brain syndrome,' or 'aging.' Instead of being left to deteriorate further, active treatment of these depressions results in a happy reawakening to life."

Treatments

The brightness of the outlook for overcoming depression stems from many developments in recent years, starting with the introduction of the first antidepressant medications in 1957 and continuing since.

A considerable array of drugs for treating depression are available today. Among them are imipramine (trade named Tofranil); desipramine (trade named Norpramin); protriptyline (trade named Vivactil); nortriptyline (trade named Aventyl); doxepin (trade named Sinequan); and amitriptyline plus perphenazine (trade named Triavil and Etrafon).

Commonly, an antidepressant can be found that may be particularly suitable for an individual patient.

No antidepressant produces dramatic overnight change. Most of the drugs take about three weeks to *begin* to work and another few weeks before the full effect starts to be felt.

Typically, the patient first begins to notice that he is becoming a little more aware of and interested in his surroundings. Not long afterward, family and friends begin to see a healthy change. And, last of all, the patients feels better.

With a few of the drugs, a diet must be observed. Certain foods and sometimes other medications are limited or eliminated because they may interact with the antidepressant and interfere with its effectiveness or cause undesirable reactions. Any patient receiving one of these drugs will receive from the physician a list of foods and drugs to be avoided. There are also certain diseases, such as one type of glaucoma, in which medications must be used with caution, and it is wise for a patient or the patient's family to provide the physician with a list of any previous illnesses.

The side effects of antidepressants are usually more annoying than serious. Dryness of the mouth and some constipation are the most common. For the first few days there may be some sleepiness and occasionally a patient may feel a bit unusual or peculiar for a short time. In some cases, there may be some dizziness or "lightheadedness," which the doctor should be informed about.

Once all depressive symptoms are gone, the medication may

be gradually reduced and then discontinued. In some cases, it may be advisable to remain on a low "maintenance" dose for a time.

Recent research indicates that for some patients who do not respond adequately to antidepressant medication, the addition of thyroid hormone to treatment may bring improvement.

In one study by Dr. F. E. Goodwin of the National Institute of Mental Health with twenty-five patients not responding well to antidepressants, fourteen improved when twenty-five micrograms of T3, a thyroid hormone, were added to treatment. In some the improvement was startlingly rapid, occurring within a few hours, but the average was five and a half days.

In another study reported by Dr. Goodwin, 75 percent of a group of patients who had been unresponsive to antidepressant agents such as Tofranil and Elavil improved rapidly when T3 was added in doses of twenty-five micrograms. The hormone was effective, Goodwin found, even though all those benefiting had apparently normal thyroid function.

Psychotherapy

Psychotherapy, when coupled with drug treatment, may be helpful. And the psychotherapy often can be brief, provided by an interested and knowledgeable family physician or internist, not necessarily by a psychiatrist. It may be simply a matter of a few short, informal talks devoted to letting the patient express his feelings and offering him support and encouragement.

Some physicians, among them Dr. Lissy Jarvik of the University of California at Los Angeles Medical Center, have been finding that group psychotherapy is particularly helpful for the elderly depressed. It may be effective for some without need for antidepressant drugs. One important aspect of group treatment for

older people is that it has social value, and many older people
are otherwise socially isolated.

A newer, quite simple form of psychotherapy, called cognitive
therapy, which is directed at helping patients through self-aware-
ness, is being used with some success.

It is based on the fact that characteristically many elderly depressed people in their daily lives talk to themselves, subvocally,
in their minds, without necessarily realizing it. They tell themselves negative things: "You're old . . . stupid . . . incapable
. . . can't expect anything." Consciously unaware of what they
are doing, they can't deal with such thoughts which reinforce
depression.

Commonly, too, the depressed have a second characteristic.
In the course of any ordinary day, most people may experience,
say, 5 to 10 percent of unpleasant moments, about the same
proportion perhaps of pleasant ones, while the rest are routine,
neither pleasant nor unpleasant. The depressed tend to completely forget the pleasant events and most of the intermediate,
remembering only the unpleasant.

In cognitive therapy, to help patients become aware of what
they are doing to themselves, they are asked to keep a daily
diary in which they record pleasant and unpleasant events as
they occur, and in which they note any automatic thoughts they
have recognized and the relationship between those thoughts
and what was going on at the time.

And in weekly hour-long sessions, patient and therapist go
over the diary and analyze the entries. Little by little, the patient
becomes aware that pleasant events do occur, and that he or
she had been selectively forgetting them before, and becomes
aware of the automatic thoughts and the misery they cause.

Cognitive therapy is in use, for example, at a newly opened
Senior Citizens Treatment Program at Long Island Jewish–Hillside Medical Center, New Hyde Park, New York.

"Often, without need for anything else, cognitive therapy

produces marked improvement within three or four months,"
says Dr. Allan Willner, who directs the program.

Sleep Deprivation Treatment

Some success is being reported, too, in the treatment of elderly
depressed patients with sleep deprivation.

The possible value of occasionally going without sleep was
first noted some years ago by European investigators. They described one depressed high school teacher who improved after
bicycling through the night; another depressed teacher who was
able to go through the examination period only after staying
awake a whole night; and a depressed physician who could manage his practice only by keeping himself awake with manual labor
every two or three nights.

Subsequently, some studies were carried out with small groups
of depressed patients who experienced a mean 35 to 40 percent
improvement in depressive symptoms after one night without
sleep. Despite the often transient effects, this form of therapy,
the investigators indicated, could produce a turn for the better
which might be maintained with antidepressant medication.

In a further study with a dozen patients, eight of whom were
suicidal, a single sleep deprivation treatment in combination
with antidepressant medication is reported to have produced a
remission of illness in six cases; in an additional three cases, a
second treatment was required for remission; and in another
case, five treatments. It was noteworthy, the investigators reported, that the patients had no difficulty staying awake except
for a critical period which usually came in the early morning
hours. After this period, there was a rather sudden lessening
of depressive symptoms.

Other more recent reports on the use of sleep deprivation
in the treatment of some 160 patients have indicated that more

than 100 (about 60 percent) responded with either brief or lasting improvement.

And not long ago, at the Douglas Hospital and McGill University in Montreal, a study was carried out with fifteen older patients, ranging in age from fifty-seven to seventy-nine, who had been suffering from depression for up to eight months.

Under medical supervision, the patients were totally deprived of sleep for a period of thirty-six hours, starting with the hour of waking on the first day, usually six to seven A.M., and continuing until six to seven P.M. of the day following the night without sleep. In most cases, sleep deprivation was used along with antidepressants.

Although it produces no miracles, sleep deprivation does look promising, report the two physicians who carried out the study, Drs. M. G. Cole and H. F. Muller. Remission occurred in six of the fifteen patients; in five as the result of deprivation plus drug therapy, in one as the result of sleep deprivation alone.

Among the patients benefiting was a seventy-eight-year-old woman who had experienced frequent depressive episodes for more than twenty-five years. When she was admitted to Douglas Hospital, she had gone through two months of drug treatment without results. On admission, she was depressed, with appetite severely diminished, and had difficulty concentrating. Further drug therapy was started in the hospital and doses were increased, but there was no improvement over a three-week period. After one thirty-six-hour sleep deprivation treatment, her mood became normal, her appetite improved, and she became active on the ward. The improvement had lasted two weeks by the time she went home from hospital, and she was still well when followed up several weeks later.

Another patient was a seventy-five-year-old woman who had had four previous depressive episodes since the death of her husband. On admission, she was mute. Relatives reported daily mood variations, loss of appetite, and insomnia. After three months of drug treatment, there was minimal improvement.

A sleep deprivation treatment had a dramatic effect. Her mood became normal, she became vivacious and talkative, and wrote letters to friends. The effect lasted only twenty-four hours. Sleep deprivation was repeated once or twice a week for a total of twelve treatments. After the second treatment, her mood improved progressively with each subsequent treatment. The final result was remission.

In general, the physicians report, sleep deprivation was well tolerated by the older patients, some of whom had heart problems.

Electroshock Therapy

In a minority of patients who do not benefit from other treatment for depression, electroshock may be used. It also may be used from the beginning in some patients whose depression is very severe, making them potentially suicidal, because shock treatment produces more immediate results.

Electroshock therapy, sometimes called ECT or EST, was first introduced in Italy in 1938 and in this country a year later. It had earlier been discovered that epileptic seizures or convulsions sometimes seemed to relieve depression. Because of the need for some means of providing relief, there was widespread use of the procedure, even though it was, to begin with, crude.

When it was first introduced, electroshock was administered without muscle relaxation and without anesthesia. It produced a powerful convulsive seizure, and several attendants were needed to hold tight to the patient during treatment in order to try to prevent bone fractures.

Later, refinements were developed. One was the use of muscle relaxants, which greatly reduced problems with fractures and sore muscles. Another consisted of sending the current through only one side of the head, which eliminated violent seizures.

Today, electroshock is markedly different from what it was originally. The patient is put gently to sleep with an intravenous anesthetic and this is followed by medication to relax muscles. Electrodes resembling headphones are then placed on the head, an electric current is applied for no more than a second, and a mild seizure is produced—minimal twitching of muscles, no "shock" of any kind.

Asleep during the treatment, the patient remains so for several minutes afterward. Then he awakens gradually and is usually up and about in fifteen to thirty minutes after the treatment is ended.

The mechanism by which electroshock relieves depression is still not understood. One theory is that somehow the current changes brain chemistry. However it works, shock treatment is often effective. Usually a patient recovers after a series of six to eight treatments.

It is not without side effects. In some, but not all, patients it produces troublesome temporary memory loss and confusion. When these effects occur, they usually clear within two or three weeks after the last treatment.

There is still controversy over shock therapy. Some physicians worry that, especially if it is used to excess, it may possibly have permanent effects on the brain, impairing memory and cognition. On the other hand, many psychiatrists consider electric shock the most effective treatment in some cases, often a lifesaver.

Is it unsafe for older people?

Says Dr. Sidney Cohen of the University of California: "Often only a few treatments suffice; an entire course is generally unnecessary. For an old patient to remain severely depressed is more dangerous than ECT."

Dr. John Romano, distinguished university professor of psychiatry at the University of Rochester, has used ECT in elderly people, including many in their mid-eighties. "Sometimes only one, two or three ECT treatments have helped old people to get better," he reports.

The Role of Lithium

There is a kind of depression which differs from what we have been talking about. The kind we have been discussing, by far the most common kind, is known as unipolar. The problem is at one pole, in one direction—down.

There is another type of depression, which is part of manic-depressive psychosis, in which mood swings are wild and uncontrolled and go from highs of great excitement to depression so deep the victim may feel suicidal. This is sometimes called bipolar depression.

In the up or manic phase, behavior is characterized by "excessive elation, hyperactivity, agitation and accelerated thinking and speaking, sometimes manifested as a flight of ideas," according to the American Psychiatric Association.

In the past, manic depression could be treated with antidepressant drugs when depression was present and electroshock and tranquilizers when mania was present. But often the mood swings would recur periodically.

Today lithium carbonate is often used. It is frequently effective in calming mania and for preventing or reducing manic episodes. The drug is of no use in overcoming a depressive episode once present; at that point an antidepressant drug is needed. But lithium is reported to help prevent the down as well as up swing when it is used in regular maintenance doses.

Is lithium of any value for *preventing* unipolar depression?

Several studies, including a four-year study at the New York State Psychiatric Institute in New York City, indicate that lithium does help to decrease episode frequency, depth of depression relapses, and duration of depressive episodes in patients who have had recurrent episodes in the past.

Lithium should be used with care under close supervision by an experienced physician. The drug's therapeutic dose and toxic dose are very close, and it is essential that any patient receiving it should have blood checks as often as every week during the first month and thereafter every month. It should not be used by patients with a history of heart or kidney disease.

Side effects may include a fine hand tremor, mild thirst, frequent urination, and diarrhea. These can often be controlled by adjustment of the dose by the physician.

A Final Word About Depression

The outlook for any depressed patient receiving adequate treatment today is excellent. There is something on the order of a 95 percent chance of returning to full functioning.

The problem, however, is recognition, especially in older people, when depression leads to distressing physical symptoms or bizarre behavior, or both, that may be dismissed as accompaniments of aging and "senility."

Ideally, anyone who feels depressed and also has physical troubles should not only seek medical help but in seeking it should mention the depressed feelings as well as body complaints.

If an elderly patient fails to do so, the next best thing is for a family member, knowing or suspecting that depression may be involved, to discuss this with the physician.

There may be observable clues, some more easily noted by a physician but some meaningful to others in the family. Indications of the possibility of depression may be found, for one thing, if the reaction of an older person to his physical troubles seems excessive considering the nature of those troubles. They may be discernible, too, when an attitude of pessimism, self-deprecation, or "giving up" is present. And they may also be found in looks of sadness, frequent sighing, slowness of movement or speech, and lack of interest in anything.

Loss is a frequent trigger of depression. But—and this is important—the loss does not have to be a major one such as the death of a loved one. Often what seems to others to be a minor event, of no real consequence, may be viewed by the depressed as a serious matter because, for whatever reason, it recalls other disappointments of the past, all of which now bulk up.

A classic example is a woman in straitened circumstances who finally managed, after many years of saving, to get together enough money to buy a piece of furniture she had long wanted. When the furniture arrived, she discovered that it was scratched. That was enough to bring on a severe depression.

10

Halting the Drug-Induced Pseudosenilities

Not long ago, a seventy-two-year-old Florida woman was hospitalized because of severe memory loss and chronic confusion. For several years, she had become increasingly unable to perform household tasks, cope with small sums of money, remember a short shopping list, find her way about indoors or along familiar streets, or recall events. She had lost all regard for the feelings of others, was given to purposeless outbursts of activity and marked emotional ups and downs, with a tendency to sexual misdemeanor.

Upon admission to the hospital, she did not recognize where she was. The results of physical examination and of many medical tests—brain scan, skull x ray, blood studies, and more—were normal.

Since suffering a heart attack fourteen years before, she had regularly taken, as prescribed, 400 milligrams of quinidine sulfate and fifty milligrams of hydrochlorothiazide daily—the former because of its ability to correct abnormal heart rhythm and the latter to help the heart by promoting excretion of excess fluids.

And her heart was fine.

But after two weeks in the hospital, she remained severely confused and disoriented and had vivid nightly hallucinations.

115

Finally, her physicians decided to discontinue the quinidine. The next day she was greatly improved. Within forty-eight hours she was well oriented for time and place and could be discharged from the hospital. A month later her memory had greatly improved, her power of concentration was markedly increased, and her personality had reverted to what it had been before she became ill.

She had been a victim of "quinidine dementia," as one of her physicians, Dr. Gordon J. Gilbert of the University of South Florida School of Medicine, Tampa, called it.

Nor is quinidine unique among otherwise helpful medications that can sometimes have undesirable effects, including behavioral changes that may mimic those of senile dementia.

Observes Dr. Gilbert: "When after thorough neurologic evaluation no cause of a progressive dementia has been established, it behooves the physician to attempt the discontinuation of any medication that has been used throughout the period of evolution of this dementia."

The value of modern medications, many of them potent, is unquestionable. But along with potential for good, they also have potential for harm.

And that harmful potential can be especially pronounced— for several reasons—among older people.

Illnesses from Drugs

Sir Hans Krebs is a world-famous scientist, a Nobel Prize winner in physiology and medicine, a member of Britain's Medical Research Council. Not long ago, Sir Hans had these pointed observations to make about modern drugs and their use:

"Side-effects of the modern highly effective drugs are almost unavoidable, because *if a drug has no side-effect then it is very likely to have no main effect either.* In other words, *no really effective drug is absolutely safe.* Usually, however, side-effects are a very minor risk, though occasionally they can become serious. Side-effects may vary from person to person, some individuals being more sensitive than others, and *what has proved safe for one person is not necessarily safe for another.*

"Known side-effects are a calculated risk. Treatment and prevention of serious diseases necessarily involve some risk. . . .

"What is of much concern [Krebs added, and the italicization is all his] *is the fact that in recent years illnesses caused by drugs have increased alarmingly, not so much on account of the inherent and calculated risks but because of excessive and unnecessary medication. This stems largely from uninformed self-medication but also from unsatisfactory management by physicians."*

Ours is commonly said to be an age of medication, a drug era, a time of "a pill for every purpose."

Whenever a check is made of the contents of household medicine cabinets, an astonishing collection comes to light. In one study by the Stanford Research Institute of households in a middle-class community in the San Francisco Bay area, the number of medications on hand was found to be as great as eighty-eight, with a mean of thirty.

Adverse drug reactions are, indeed, a major public health problem. In 1973, Dr. Kenneth L. Melmon of the University of California Medical Center, San Francisco, found that 3 to 5 percent of all admissions to the hospitals under study were due to illnesses caused by drugs. In testimony before a Senate subcommittee, experts estimated that 1,500,000 hospital admissions a year are the result of adverse drug reactions, about 80 percent of which come from prescribed and about 20 percent from non-prescribed drugs.

One Part of the Problem

Too few patients understand very much—often, anything at all—about the drugs they take. Because they are incapable of understanding? Perhaps in a very few cases. Often they may not receive adequate information.

In one recent study of patients taking prescribed drugs at home, over 83 percent were found to be in possible danger because they knew so little about the drugs. Almost three-fourths of the patients did not know of *any* symptoms at all that might indicate harmful side effects of their medicines.

For lack of understanding, patients may not take the proper dosages of drugs. Digitalis is a valuable heart drug, but it can be useless when dosage is inadequate and can cause serious disturbances when dosage is excessive. Yet a University of California study found that the average outpatient has a 95 percent probability of taking anywhere between 40 percent and 140 percent of a prescribed regimen of digitalis.

One study of more than 300 patients being treated by forty-six physicians in a Midwestern city found that the patients were failing to take 19 percent of the drugs prescribed, taking 19 to 20 percent more drugs than the doctors had ordered, and timing drugs incorrectly in 17 percent of the cases.

Why? "When patients were informed as to what was expected of them, their behaviors conformed to that expectation more than 85 percent of the time. The major problem was communication," according to the study published in the *American Journal of Public Health.*

Why the communication problem? One reason can be physician busyness—an excessive patient load.

But many physicians seem to believe that what a patient doesn't know won't hurt him. Does this have any basis in fact? Recently, when the Given Health Center in Burlington, Vermont, took an unusual step, giving all of its 8000 patients copies of their medical records, 93 percent of the patients said anxiety about their health was reduced.

Another factor often involved is the "medical mystique." About that, the professional journal *The New Physician* has observed: "It feeds on a system that makes young people suffer and sacrifice to enter its highest rank, at each step becoming more convinced that if they make it to the top, they sure as hell will be gods. It is a system wherein hundreds of thousands of concerned, intelligent Americans allow information about their health, their lives, their bodies to be kept from them or dispensed only in little bits at the discretion of their doctors."

To be fair, patients are not always blameless for poor communication.

They may be told things by their physicians that they don't understand and fail to ask for clarification. Some don't want to appear to be stupid; some, aware of a waiting room full of patients, don't want to take up the physician's time; some fear they may seem to be questioning the physician's judgment. As a result, they go home confused—and often needlessly worried and anxious.

Nor do prescription labels necessarily provide all the information needed.

When University of Rochester Medical Center investigators carried out a special study on how patients interpreted instructions on each of ten prescription labels, they discovered that *not once* was a label uniformly interpreted by all patients.

One prescription, for example, called for taking penicillin G three times a day and at bedtime. The vast majority—89.5 percent—of patients took this to mean they should use the drug with meals and at bedtime. But some drugs—and penicillin G is one—should be taken on an empty stomach to facilitate their absorption and effective activity.

Reported the investigators: "We discovered a surprisingly wide range of interpretations, a high frequency of misinterpretations, and a significant potential for failure or illness as a consequence of mistaken interpretations."

They urged physicians to provide better instructions on how to take medication and to review the instructions with patients.

And what of the patient knowing the names of all medications prescribed for him? Should labels indicate names as well as prescription numbers and directions?

More and more physicians are coming to believe so. But not all specifically instruct pharmacists to label.

Under the heading of "Chromoconfusion," one recent medical report in the *Canadian Medical Association Journal* called attention to the problem.

Suppose, as an example, it suggested to physicians, that you are treating a patient suffering from severe high blood pressure, mild anginal chest pain, hyperuricemia (elevated uric acid levels in the blood), mild diabetes, and congestive heart failure. And suppose, it also suggested, that you happen to prescribe these drugs, all justified for treating various aspects of the poor patient's many ailments: Lanoxin, Hygroton, Isordil, Ismelin, Serpasil, Zyloprim, and DBI.

The prescriptions are not labeled, and these happen to be all "little white pills"—which is the only way the patient can refer to them.

"Try to envision," the Canadian report proposed, "how to ask your patient, the next time he comes to your office, how compliant he is about taking the 'little round white pill for the heart,' the 'little round white pill for water,' the 'little white round pill for blood pressure,' and the 'little round white pill for angina.' If he brings the pills with him, just think how you will be confused; if he does not bring the pills with him, just imagine your frustrating conversation about all those 'little white round pills.' Unknowingly, you have now become a little-round-white-pill doctor. And we would not be surprised if some of your clientele would not develop decompensated heart failure, digitalis intoxication, uncontrolled hypertension, orthostat hypotension, etc."

Naming drugs on labels can be valuable for helping avoid mistakes in taking medication. If undesirable side effects occur or if there should be an accidental overdose, immediate identification of the medication could help prevent fatality. And a patient's knowledge of what he or she is taking can be valuable if another physician has to be consulted while on a trip or when the physician is away.

Another Part of the Problem:
Many Rx's vs. Real Medical Attention

Concerned about the drug prescribing practices of some physicians, Drs. Peter P. Lamy of the University of Maryland and Robert E. Vestal of Vanderbilt University not long ago cited a case illustrative of what may be no rare problem.

An elderly woman had high blood pressure, congestive heart failure, diabetes, and ankle swelling, and was obese. Her physician had prescribed a reducing diet plus a drug for her diabetes; plus Peritrate and nitroglycerin for her heart; plus a diuretic for her elevated blood pressure; plus antacids for her vague complaints about stomach upsets.

Were all the drugs justified? Probably only two were, Drs. Lamy and Vestal pointed out.

The diuretic was appropriate for both her congestive heart failure and high blood pressure but could make treatment of her diabetes more difficult. In that case, insulin rather than an oral antidiabetes drug should have been considered; although, in fact, her diabetic problem might well have diminished or disappeared altogether if she had lost weight.

Unfortunately, the woman had not been led to understand clearly the importance of her diet, or even the details of the diet, and had not followed it. She continued to overeat, and her physician continued to treat her stomach symptoms with antacids. Both Peritrate and nitroglycerin had been prescribed only because of a vague complaint that her chest hurt. Taking the diuretic only erratically, she had little benefit from it.

"In ten years," Drs. Lamy and Vestal noted, "the physician

has not changed the regimen at all, even though lack of success should have prompted review and change. It would have been far better for the physician to have taken the time to explain the need for adhering to the diet, to make sure the diuretic was taken as directed, and to consider whether the chest pain merited any drug therapy at all. Our conclusion is that in this patient drug prescribing has replaced real medical attention."

Drugs and the Elderly

The elderly use a disproportionate share of drugs. While making up 10 percent of the population, people over sixty-five consume 25 percent of all prescription drugs, according to recent studies. And there is no reason to believe that the proportions are any different for nonprescription agents.

Given the disproportionately heavy use, it could be expected that there might be a certain amount of misuse and other problems. But the amount has finally become of deep concern among experts on the care of the elderly.

It was that concern which led to a national symposium at the University of Miami which focused on drug problems in older people.

All aspects of those problems were considered. Obviously enough, older people more often than younger ones have several disorders for which drugs may be needed. But participants in the symposium also noted that problems arise because many of the elderly tend to hoard old drugs, share medications with neighbors, use duplicate medications prescribed by different physicians, mix different drugs in one container, and often get confused by poor instructions and microscopic labels they would not be able to understand even if they could make them out.

The symposium emphasized that the elderly will probably remain at high risk until new attitudes about drug prescribing and management are adopted by physicians, pharmacists, nurses, and others concerned with care of older people.

Moreover, physicians and patients and their families need to recognize a frequently overlooked fact: that people over sixty-five are in much greater danger of unfavorable drug reactions—and not only because more drugs are prescribed for them.

When they get into the bodies of older people, drugs "have quite a mind of their own," pointed out Dr. Eric Pfeiffer of the University of Colorado.

In older people, drugs don't necessarily act the way the book says they will act. And that is partly because drugs are traditionally tested only in young people, who have a single disease, are taking only one medication, and are otherwise healthy.

In addition, older people often have reduced metabolic activity, which means that a little drug can go a long way, that dosage should not necessarily be the standard dosage used for younger people, that it may have to be lower, even only half the standard dosage, if it is to work without producing undesirable reactions.

Moreover, excretion rates in older people may be lower than in younger people, which means that drugs are retained in the body longer, and unless this is taken into account, overdosage is likely.

As discussion throughout the symposium indicated, present medical textbooks unfortunately contain no specific information on how physicians should prescribe for older people. They contain no information on how to counter patients' expectations that unless a drug is prescribed a physician hasn't earned his fee. They do not emphasize that one of the most critical errors made by physicians in treating older people is the assumption that other physicians have not been, or even at the moment are not, treating them too and that their older patients are not already taking medications.

Many of the authorities participating in the symposium stated that it can be vital with any patient, and especially an older patient, to make him or her a partner in the drug-taking regimen.

Dr. Pfeiffer emphasized that the physician should explain what a drug is all about and should try to make the regimen as simple as possible. He should understand that the older person usually requires less of any given drug than a younger or even middle-aged person. And if there is to be a rule, it should be fewer doses, fewer pills, and more memory devices to help patients to remember when to take medication.

"If we can provide dialpaks for the young, intelligent, highly motivated woman, why not for the elderly?" Pfeiffer argued.

It's incumbent upon physicians, too, symposium participants pointed out, to recognize that many older people do not see and hear as well as they used to, and should be spoken to more distinctly. Rapid-fire prescribing instructions such as "Two of these in the morning and bedtime, and three of these after each meal"—which can be difficult even for younger people to keep straight—may be even more so for older people.

It is incumbent upon physicians, too, to make the patient feel willing to assert himself if he doesn't understand what the drug is supposed to do or anything about it. And the patient should be prepared not only for what a drug is supposed to do but also what side reactions it may cause.

If the recommendations coming from the symposium were heeded by all physicians, almost certainly older patients would have fewer seriously troublesome reactions from drugs, including those mimicking symptoms of dementia.

DRUGS THAT MAY PRODUCE
SENILITY-LIKE SYMPTOMS

Many symptoms that may seem like those of senility can be produced by drugs.

Such symptoms include:

Agitation
Anxiety

Disturbed Concentration
Confusion
Delusions
Depression
Disorientation
Euphoria
Excitement
Shuffling or unsteady gait
Hallucinations
Irritability
Mental acuity impairment
Nervousness
Nightmares
Restlessness
Speech slurring
Urinary incontinence

The following are commonly used drugs that can in some people produce one or more such symptoms.

AN IMPORTANT NOTE ABOUT SIDE EFFECTS

Although drugs can produce undesirable reactions, they do so in only a small minority of users, usually in less than 5 percent, often in less than 1 percent.

When side effects do occur, they may do so because of inappropriate dosage or because of an unusual sensitivity to a particular drug in an individual.

Side effects can be peculiar. Some may develop when a drug is first used and may be mild and may disappear before long as the drug is continued. Others may be mild or severe and may not disappear.

Many people accept side effects as a price to be paid for treatment, when, in fact, a change of dosage or a change to another medication equally good for the purpose may eliminate them.

In many cases, too, people suffering drug symptoms are unaware that they come from medication, believing that they may be additional symptoms of the original problem.

A knowledge of what symptoms particular drugs may produce can be useful. It should not be scary.

If there should be any suspicion that disturbing symptoms are coming from a drug, it should be discussed with a physician without delay. Almost certainly, he can help in one way or another—either using measures which may counter the symptoms or providing reassurance that the disturbances will be only fleeting.

Drugs in the following pages are listed in alphabetical order according to trade name. For each, the generic name is also listed in parentheses, followed by the purpose of the drug and the symptom or symptoms it may sometimes produce which may mimic those of senility.

Aldactazide (spironolactone with hydrochlorothiazide). For edema, high blood pressure.
Restlessness, confusion.
Aldactone (spironolactone). For edema, high blood pressure.
Confusion.
Aldomet (methyldopa). For high blood pressure.
Mental acuity decrease.
Aldoril (methyldopa with hydrochlorothiazide). For high blood pressure.
Depression, mental acuity decrease, nightmares, restlessness.
Ambenyl Expectorant (codeine, bromodiphenhydramine, diphenhydramine, ammonium chloride, potassium guaiacolsulfonate, menthol). For cough.
Nervousness, restlessness, confusion.
Apresoline (hydralazine). For high blood pressure.
Anxiety, depression, disorientation.
Artane (trihexyphenidyl). For parkinsonism (shaking palsy) and control of some nervous system side effects of tranquilizers.
Nervousness.

Azo Gantrisin (sulfisoxazole, phenazopyridine). For painful urinary infections.
Depression, hallucinations.
Benadryl (diphenhydramine). For allergy, motion sickness, insomnia.
Confusion, restlessness.
Bendectin (dicyclomine, doxylamine, pyridoxine). For nausea and vomiting.
Irritability.
Bentyl (dicyclomine). For irritable bowel, intestinal inflammation.
Nervousness.
Butazolidin and *Butazolidin Alka* (phenylbutazone). For arthritic conditions, gout, painful shoulder.
Agitation, confusion.
Chlor-Trimeton (chlorpheniramine maleate). For allergy.
Nervousness.
Compazine (prochlorperazine). For severe nausea, anxiety, tension, agitation.
Agitation, shuffling gait.
Dalmane (flurazepam). For insomnia.
Confusion, disorientation, hallucinations, irritability, nervousness, restlessness, speech slurring.
Darvon (propoxyphene); Darvon Compound-65 (with aspirin, phenacetin, caffeine); Darvon-N with ASA (with aspirin); Darvocet-N (with acetaminophen). For mild to moderate pain.
Euphoria, restlessness.
Demerol (meperidine). Narcotic for pain.
Agitation, disorientation, euphoria, hallucinations, restlessness.
Dilantin (phenytoin). For epilepsy.
Confusion, nervousness, speech slurring.
Dimetane (brompheniramine). For allergy.
Confusion, euphoria, excitement, nervousness, restlessness.
Diupres (chlorothiazide and reserpine). For high blood pressure.

Depression, nervousness, nightmares, restlessness.

Diuril (chlorothiazide). For edema, high blood pressure.

Restlessness.

Doriden (glutethimide). For insomnia.

Excitement.

Drixoral (dexbrompheniramine and d-isoephedrine). For nasal congestion.

Confusion, restlessness, anxiety.

Elavil (amitriptyline). For depression.

Anxiety, disturbed concentration, confusion, disorientation, excitement, hallucinations, nightmares, restlessness.

Equanil (meprobamate). For anxiety, tension.

Euphoria, excitement, speech slurring.

Esidrix (hydrochlorothiazide). For high blood pressure, edema.

Restlessness.

Etrafon (perphenazine and amitriptyline). For anxiety, agitation, depressed mood.

Anxiety, confusion, delusions, excitement, urinary incontinence.

Gantanol (sulfamethoxazole). For infections.

Depression, hallucinations.

Gantrisin (sulfisoxazole). For infections.

Depression, hallucinations.

HydroDIURIL (hydrochlorothiazide). For edema.

Restlessness.

Hydropres (hydrochlorothiazide and reserpine). For high blood pressure.

Anxiety, depression, nervousness, nightmares.

Hygroton (chlorthalidone). For high blood pressure, edema.

Restlessness.

Inderal (propranolol). For angina pectoris, heart rhythm abnormality, pheochromocytoma, high blood pressure.

Depression, hallucinations.

Indocin (indomethacin). For arthritic conditions.

Confusion, depression.

Ionamin (phentermine resin). For weight reduction.

Euphoria, restlessness.

Isordil (isosorbide dinitrate). For angina pectoris.

Restlessness.

Kaon (potassium gluconate). For correcting low blood potassium levels.

Confusion.

Librax (chlordiazepoxide and clidinium bromide). For relief of gastrointestinal symptoms.

Confusion.

Librium (chlordiazepoxide). For anxiety, tension.

Confusion.

Lomotil (diphenoxylate with atropine). For diarrhea.

Depression, euphoria, restlessness.

Marax (ephedrine sulfate, theophylline, hydroxyzine). For asthma.

Excitement, unsteady gait, nervousness.

Mellaril (thioridazine). For psychiatric disorders.

Agitation, confusion, excitement, restlessness, urinary incontinence.

Meprobamate (this is the generic name). For anxiety, tension.

Confusion, euphoria, excitement, speech slurring.

Nembutal (pentobarbital). For insomnia, sedation.

Excitement.

Noludar (methyprylon). For insomnia.

Excitement.

Norgesic (orphenadrine, methylbenzhydryl, aspirin, phenacetin, caffeine). For pain.

Confusion.

Ornade (chlorpheniramine, phenylpropanolamine, isopropamide). For nasal congestion.

Irritability, nervousness.

Percodan (oxycodone, aspirin, phenacetin, caffeine). For pain.

Euphoria, restlessness.

Periactin (cyproheptadine). For allergies.

Confusion, euphoria, excitement, hallucinations, restlessness.

Peritrate (pentaerythritol). For angina pectoris.

Restlessness.

Phenobarbital (this is generic name). For sedation.

Excitement.

Polaramine (dexchlorpheniramine). For allergies.

Nervousness, restlessness.

Pro-Banthīne (propantheline). For peptic ulcer.

Nervousness.

Proloid (thyroglobulin). For low thyroid function.

From overdosage: nervousness.

Quinidine sulfate (this is generic name). For heart rhythm abnormalities.

Confusion, excitement.

Rauzide (rauwolfia, bendroflumethiazide). For high blood pressure.

Anxiety, depression, nervousness.

Regroton (chlorthalidone and reserpine). For high blood pressure.

Depression, nightmares, restlessness.

Reserpine (this is generic name). For high blood pressure.

Anxiety, depression, nightmares.

Ritalin (methylphenidate). For mild depression, apathetic or withdrawn senile behavior.

Nervousness.

Salutensin (hydroflumethiazide and reserpine). For high blood pressure.

Anxiety, nervousness, nightmares, restlessness.

Seconal (sodium secobarbital). For insomnia.

Excitement.

Ser-Ap-Es (reserpine, hydralazine, hydrochlorothiazide). For high blood pressure.

Anxiety, depression, disorientation, nervousness, nightmares, restlessness.

Serax (oxazepam). For anxiety, tension, agitation, irritability.

Disorientation, euphoria, hallucinations, speech slurring.

Sinequan (doxepin). For anxiety, depression.

Confusion, disorientation, hallucinations.

Stelazine (trifluoperazine). For anxiety, tension, agitation, psychotic disorders.

Agitation.

Sterazolidin (phenylbutazone, prednisone, aluminum hydroxide, magnesium trisilicate). For arthritis, bursitis, gout, acute fibrositis.

Agitation.

Synthroid (sodium levothyroxine). For thyroid deficiency.

From overdosage: nervousness.

Talwin (pentazocine). For moderate to severe pain.

Euphoria, excitement, hallucinations.

Tandearil (oxyphenbutazone). For arthritis, gout, painful shoulder, some other inflammatory conditions.

Agitation, confusion.

Tenuate (diethylpropion). For weight reduction.

Anxiety, depression, euphoria, nervousness, restlessness.

Thyroid (generic name). For thyroid deficiency.

With excessive dosage: nervousness.

Tigan (trimethobenzamide). For nausea and vomiting.

Depression, disorientation.

Tofranil (imipramine). For depression.

Agitation, anxiety, confusion, delusions, disorientation, hallucinations, nightmares, restlessness.

Tranxene (clorazepate). For anxiety.

Confusion, depression, irritability, nervousness, speech slurring.

Triaminic (phenylpropanolamine, pheniramine, pyrilamine). For nasal congestion, postnasal drip.

Nervousness.

Triavil (perphenazine, amitriptyline). For anxiety and/or depression.

Agitation, anxiety, disturbed consciousness, confusion, delusions, disorientation, excitement, hallucinations, restlessness.

Tuinal (secobarbital and amobarbital). For insomnia.
  Excitement.
Tuss-Ornade (caramiphen, chlorpheniramine, phenylpropanol-
amine). For cough, upper respiratory congestion, excessive nasal
secretion.
  Irritability, nervousness.
Valium (diazepam). For tension, anxiety, muscle spasm.
  Anxiety, confusion, depression, speech slurring, urinary incon-
tinence.

PRACTICAL GUIDELINES
ON DRUG TAKING

Drug–Drug Interactions

Older people often take more than a single drug. When two
or more drugs are used, each may work effectively without interfering with the other. Sometimes one may even help the other.

But it is also possible for use of one drug on top of another
to be potentially harmful. One may interfere with the activity
of the other, making it useless. Or the second drug may make
it necessary to reduce or raise the dosage of the first to avoid
problems.

Consider, for example, a patient who was hospitalized because
of a heart attack, made a good recovery, but ten days after coming
home developed an alarming condition.

While in the hospital, he had been given anticoagulant medication as a precaution against blood clotting after the heart attack.
At home, as directed, he continued to take the anticoagulant.
But now the drug was thinning his blood excessively and he
was in danger of fatal hemorrhaging.

Why the change in the drug's effects? It turned out that while
in the hospital he had been given phenobarbital upon retiring
at night. The sedative, in the course of its metabolism or handling
in the body, stimulated liver chemicals that broke down the anti-

coagulant faster. At home, without the sedative, the anticoagulant activity continued longer and was more potent. Without the sedative, the patient now was getting in effect an overdose of anticoagulant. The problem, once understood, was quickly solved with a change in anticoagulant dosage.

Only recently have many important drug interactions been observed, and the list is growing rapidly. In fact, understanding—and taking into account—interactions between drugs is coming to be virtually a new science in medicine.

Some further examples of interactions:

Aspirin or an aspirinlike compound (salicylate) is available not only in tablets but as an ingredient of other nonprescription preparations for headaches and other aches and pains, and for colds and fever. It is also present in some over-the-counter sleeping tablets and other readily available combinations. Aspirin and other salicylates can interact with anticoagulant drugs to bring on bleeding and they can decrease the effectiveness of some drugs taken for gout.

Many nonprescription nose drops and sprays; decongestant medicines for coughs, sinusitis, and colds; and prescription drugs used to reduce appetite contain ingredients known as sympathomimetic amines. These can counteract the effects of drugs used to lower high blood pressure. They can also cause a dangerous increase in blood pressure in people taking certain drugs for depression, especially those known as MAO inhibitors, which include Parnate, Marplan, and Nardil. These and other MAO inhibitors—including the antibiotic Furoxone and Eutonyl, a drug used for high blood pressure—interact similarly with tyramine, a compound in aged cheeses and Chianti wines.

If a patient is taking an antidepressant drug such as amitriptyline and is also given guanethidine for high blood pressure, the amitriptyline nullifies the pressure-lowering activity of guanethidine. If a patient is taking an antihistamine for allergy and consumes alcohol, central nervous system depression may sometimes follow.

Nose drops and related medications may tend to cause irregular heartbeats, but when they are taken with digitalis, heartbeat irregularity is far more likely.

For any patient, and certainly an elderly one, the best means of protection against potentially dangerous drug interactions is to let any physician consulted about a new condition know what, if any, drugs already are being used, both prescription drugs and ordinary over-the-counter drugs such as aspirin or other pain relievers, antacids, laxatives, and the like. It also is advisable to ask a physician when he prescribes a drug whether it will be all right if necessary to take aspirin or other agents.

Drug–Diet Interactions

Recently it has become clear that long-term use of some valuable drugs can sometimes affect nutrition.

Some reduce appetite at the risk of inadequate nutrition; others induce malabsorption, interfering with the body's absorption of nutrients from food.

Among drugs that may interfere with nutrient absorption are phenolphthalein, a common laxative; methotrexate, sometimes used for severe psoriasis; and colchicine, used for gout.

Some oral antidiabetic agents may interfere with absorption of vitamin B_{12}. High intakes of L-dopa, a valuable drug for shaking palsy, may cause vitamin B_6 deficiency. Some drugs such as methotrexate can cause deficiency of the vitamin folic acid. Other drugs can lead to vitamin deficiencies by greatly increasing requirements. For example, phenobarbital and a related compound, primidone, and the antiepilepsy agent Dilantin seem to increase the turnover in the body of vitamin D so that more is needed to fill normal requirements.

Drug-caused nutritional deficiencies can be prevented. If a drug must be taken for control of a chronic disease over long periods, a responsible physician can see to it that the patient receives necessary additional vitamins or other nutrients in the diet or as dietary supplements.

Not only may some drugs impair food absorption; some foods may impair drug absorption. Some drugs are best taken on an empty stomach; some at other times; and some should never be taken with particular foods.

A recent report on drug and diet interactions offers these useful guidelines:

To be taken on an empty stomach (two to three hours before meals):
   benzathine penicillin G
   cloxacillin (Tegopen)
   erythromycin
   lincomycin (Lincocin)
   methacycline (Rondomycin)
   phenoxymethyl penicillin (penicillin V)
   tetracycline antibiotics (except Declomycin which can upset
      the stomach)

To be taken one half hour before meals:
   belladonna and its alkaloids
   Librax
   Donnatal
   Ritalin
   Pyridium
   Preludin
   Pro-Banthine

To be taken with meals or food:
   aminophylline
   antidiabetes drugs
   APC (aspirin, phenacetin, caffeine)
   Diuril, HydroDIURIL
   Dilantin
   Ponstel
   Flagyl

Furadantin, Macrodantin
prednisone
prednisolone
Serpasil
reserpine
Dyrenium
Artane
Temaril

Not to be taken with milk:
Dulcolax
potassium chloride
potassium iodide
tetracycline antibiotics except Vibramycin

Not to be taken with fruit juices:
ampicillin
benzathine penicillin G
cloxacillin
erythromycin

Alcohol to be avoided while taking:
Dymelor
antihistamines
chloral hydrate
Librium
Diabinese
Lomotil
MAO inhibitor antidepressants (Marplan, Parnate, Eutonyl,
    Nardil)
Antivert
Quaalude
Flagyl
narcotics
Orinase

MAKING MEDICINE
MORE HELPFUL, LESS HARMFUL

In a recent special report in the *New York State Journal of Medicine*, Dr. M. R. P. Hall, a professor of geriatic medicine, noted that "many geriatricians cynically claim that their greatest therapeutic successes are achieved by stopping the drugs with which their colleagues were poisoning their patients."

That is certainly not to deny what is a fact: that modern drugs are valuable when they are really needed, properly prescribed, consumed only as long as needed, and then with whatever safeguards may be needed to reduce to the barest minimum any possibility of undesirable reactions.

But it is also a fact that there is a tremendous overconsumption of drugs, a haste for many patients to demand a pill, willy-nilly, when it is not really essential—when other measures such as improvement of diet and perhaps of one or more living habits could be used more effectively. And, against their better judgment, some physicians give in to the irrational demand; and, no less unfortunately, some physicians substitute medicines for good medical care.

It's a fact, too, that not all drugs prescribed need to be used continuously. Many serve a valuable immediate purpose and thereafter are unnecessary. Digitalis, for example, is a very important drug for heart problems. Yet at least one recent study found that continuous treatment with digitalis may be unnecessary in about 70 percent of cases.

For anyone taking drugs—and especially for an older person who may be taking several—a periodic review of their need by the treating physician is certainly advisable.

And anyone taking drugs—and especially an older person—would be well advised to be knowledgeable about their use, to be less assertive in demanding still another medication and more assertive, if necessary, in demanding from physicians information on all the points suggested in this chapter: Why is a particular drug being used? What is its purpose? What can be expected of it and when? What are the potential side effects that are likely to be hazardous and should be reported back to the physician without delay? What, if anything, can be done to minimize the likelihood of side effects developing? Do all the drugs being taken go well together? And what possible drug–diet interactions may occur and how can they be overcome or compensated for?

11

Overcoming the
Deficiency-Triggered

A few years ago, a British investigator reported striking results of a study with a group of elderly patients admitted to a hospital in Sheffield. Over a period of six months, 254 patients were admitted to the hospital's geriatric unit.

For the study, Dr. M. L. Mitra chose only elderly patients with confusional states. And he was able to demonstrate that the confusion in many was linked to simple, measurable vitamin deficiencies and often disappeared when the deficiencies were corrected.

These were some typical patients:

- A sixty-six-year-old woman was admitted because of a confusional state and deterioration in gait and mobility. Among the tests performed were some for possible vitamin deficiencies. After two weeks of treatment with a concentrated solution of vitamin B complex, her confusional state cleared, mobility and gait improved, and she could be discharged home.
- An eighty-eight-year-old woman who lived alone and ran her own lodging house was admitted because of severe dehydration and a confusional state. On physical examination, the only abnormality detected was blood in the stools. To make up for the blood loss, she received transfusions. X-

ray examination of the gastrointestinal tract showed nothing abnormal. Liver function tests, however, did show abnormalities—which turned out to be related to a drug she had been taking at home for the confusional state. After the drug was stopped and liver function values returned to normal, tests revealed need for vitamin B complex. She soon regained her mental faculties.

• An eighty-nine-year-old woman living with her daughter was admitted on recommendation of her physicians for investigation of anemia and an abdominal mass. The mass was found to be a distended bladder and disappeared when the bladder was emptied via a catheter. But the patient was very confused and severely dehydrated. Her anemia was due to iron deficiency, but studies showed plenty of iron in her blood and an inability to utilize it properly. Tests also showed B complex deficiency. On receiving B complex, her confusional state improved greatly. And her anemia was helped by an iron supplement and a small amount of the vitamin folic acid.

• A seventy-two-year-old woman who lived alone was admitted for what her doctor believed to be congestive heart failure and kidney failure. On admission, she was confused; she also showed a pattern of skin pigmentation which had been attributed to sunbathing but was classic for pellagra, a deficiency of the B vitamin niacin. The pellagra diagnosis was confirmed by tests. On vitamin treatment, she became a different woman and when discharged home was normal except for some osteoarthritis of the knees.

• An eighty-four-year-old woman, admitted to hospital for acute exacerbation of chronic bronchitis, also was confused and had bone tenderness and multiple bruises, both of the latter suggesting vitamin C deficiency. The deficiency was confirmed. In addition to treatment for the bronchitis, she received a gram of vitamin C daily for two weeks. Upon discharge, she was free of confusion, bone tenderness, and bruises.

A Surprising Incidence

Nobody knows precisely to what extent mental and physical declines in older people may be due to malnutrition, but in many cases it could be a substantial contributing factor.

Nor need the malnutrition be severe to make its contribution. Much recent research indicates that mental and behavioral disturbances can result from marginal deficiencies and that marginal deficiencies are far from rare.

In the mid-1960s, studies in Syracuse and Onondaga County, New York, among two groups in the population—adolescents and the elderly—found inadequacies of vitamins A, B_1, and C.

Later these findings were confirmed and extended to the whole country by nutritional status surveys by various federal government agencies, including a U.S. Department of Agriculture Market Basket Survey of 1965; a Department of Health, Education, and Welfare Ten State Nutrition Survey completed in 1972; and a more recent Health and Nutrition Examination Survey by the Department of Health, Education, and Welfare.

The Ten State Survey, for example, covered 83,000 persons. It found that one-fourth of those living below the poverty level were anemic because of insufficient iron in their diets. The diets of 8 percent of poverty-level persons proved to be low or deficient in vitamin A. Seven percent were deficient in vitamin C, and 17 percent in vitamin B_2.

The Ten State Survey also found deficiencies in about 8 percent of better-off Americans. And it discovered that persons over sixty in all income levels and ethnic groups showed signs of general undernutrition.

In another more recent survey, the U.S. Department of Agriculture found that in some age groups, regardless of income level, the average intake for several vital nutrients—calcium, iron, magnesium, and vitamin B_6—was below recommended levels.

In hospital studies, deficiencies among patients have been

found to be surprisingly common. Not long ago, the University of Cape Town, South Africa, set up a special clinical nutrition research unit to help physicians diagnose nutritional diseases in complicated cases. When the unit looked, first, for thiamine deficiency in hospital patients, carefully blood-testing for the vitamin, it found 43 percent of patients deficient. In some cases, alcoholism was a presumptive cause; in many others, peptic ulcer, gastroenteritis, or malabsorption was involved.

In 1974, investigators checking the status of 599 expectant American mothers for thiamine found more than 25 percent deficient.

In various studies in the United States and by the World Health Organization elsewhere, deficiency of another vitamin, folic acid, has been found in one-third to one-half of all pregnant women.

In a British study of fifty-nine elderly psychiatric patients newly admitted to hospital, forty-eight had subnormal folic acid levels. In another study, low levels of folic acid were discovered in thirty-seven of seventy-five psychiatric patients. And in a University of Illinois study in 1977, older people with such symptoms as forgetfulness, apathy, depression, and psychosis often turned out to have low blood levels of folic acid.

Because of evidence indicating that many American diets today are deficient in a whole series of ten important nutrients—vitamin A, thiamine, riboflavin, niacin, B_6, folic acid, iron, calcium, magnesium, and zinc—the National Research Council's Food and Nutrition Board recently has been urging that many foods be enriched with these materials.

Special Problems in Older People

For more than one reason, nutritional problems in the population as a whole may be magnified in older people.

Low or marginal income may be responsible in some cases. Lack of interest in eating because of loneliness is not uncommon.

Food faddism, too, is an important determinant of the diet of many older people searching for relief from various ailments and heeding the call of quack elixirs.

Malnutrition may accentuate appetite loss in older people. By making them feel weak and ill, it not only may perpetuate but even accelerate itself.

Moreover, aging, to the extent that it is accompanied by a reduction of physical activity, brings with it a reduced overall need for food—but not for food values. Actually, older people need more food value per unit of food than younger people who have larger food intakes. But often they do not get such value.

And various disorders in older people may tend to decrease the absorption of some vitamins and other nutrients and thereby may increase requirements for them.

Testifying in 1977 before the Senate Committee on Nutrition and Human Needs, Dr. Robert N. Butler, director of the National Institute on Aging, noted: "The aged patient is a major user of drugs. There is evidence that, like variations in nutritional needs, drug responses in the elderly are also different from those of young adults. It can reasonably be assumed that interactions of drugs and nutrition have special relevance for the elderly. For example, deficiencies in fat-soluble vitamins such as A, D, and E in the aged are frequently due to interference in absorption caused by the habitual use of the common laxative mineral oil, which drains away fat-soluble vitamins.

"In addition, various drugs used in the treatment of chronic diseases are known to interfere with the absorption or utilization of specific nutrients, including vitamin B_{12} and folic acid. The possible synergistic effect of a borderline nutrient intake with prolonged drug therapy in the older adult may also be a fruitful area of investigation. . . . Understanding the interaction between nutrition and exercise in the aged is also important. It may not be possible to obtain adequate nutrition and maintain a desirable body weight without some exercise."

And Dr. Butler had another point to emphasize:

"One of the major impacts of diet in old age is its effect on cerebral functioning, mood and behavior. Research on this topic is just beginning, but it holds the promise of important discoveries in the future. For example, malnutrition and associated anemia are two of the primary causes of reversible brain syndrome. Reversible brain syndrome is characterized by fluctuating levels of awareness which may vary from mild confusion to stupor or active delirium. The patient is typically disoriented, mistaking one person for another, and may have other intellectual functions impaired as well. These and other symptoms mimic those of chronic and irreversible brain syndromes and may therefore be misdiagnosed as such and left untreated. If handled as the true medical emergencies they are, reversible brain syndromes often respond well to treatment. However, untreated reversible brain syndromes can quickly become chronic and irreversible. The personal anguish and costs of unnecessary institutionalization are severe for those whose reversible brain syndromes are not correctly diagnosed and treated."

The Stages of Deficiency

Nutritional deficiencies and the manifestations that accompany them do not develop suddenly. Rather, they go through a series of stages which recently have been identified.

To begin with, a nutrient may be in short supply for any of several possible reasons—inadequate intake in the diet, a malabsorption disorder that interferes with the nutrient's entry into the body even if it is present in adequate amounts in the diet, or interference with the body's actual utilization of the nutrient as the result of the actions of a drug.

In this first stage, whatever stores of the nutrient there have been in body tissues are gradually diminished. And if this continues, the tissue stores may be so reduced as to retard any biochemical activities in the body for which the nutrient is needed.

In the next stage, the biochemical retardation reaches a point at which behavioral changes begin to become manifest—appetite loss, general malaise, irritability, sleeping difficulty.

In a subsequent stage, as the deficiency progresses, behavioral changes are accentuated; and now, in addition, physical changes may become apparent—leg swelling, pain on walking, or other problems depending upon the particular nutrient deficiency.

SPECIFIC DEFICIENCIES

Thiamine (Vitamin B$_1$)

At the University of Minnesota some years ago, Dr. J. Brozek investigated the psychological effects of thiamine deficiency. Working with young men, all normal to begin with, he used standard psychological tests to determine any changes that might occur as the men were deprived of adequate thiamine intake.

Brozek found large changes in the direction of deterioration on the psychoneurotic scales of the Minnesota Multiphasic Personality Inventory, and later found that these changes could be reversed with thiamine supplements. Significantly, too, the study established that personality changes appeared before such other symptoms as gastric distress, weight loss, and abnormal tingling and burning sensations that thiamine deficiency may produce.

Other studies have shown that disturbances associated with thiamine deficiency may include irritability, memory impairment, depression, difficulty in concentrating, and confusion. Such manifestations, of course, can come from problems other than thiamine deficiency; but when they are associated with the deficiency, they clear up readily with administration of thiamine.

Heavy alcohol intake may lead to thiamine deficiency by inter-ferring with normal absorption of the vitamin. But the deficiency can affect non-drinkers.

Although the daily adult requirement is small—in the range of one to one and a half milligrams—so is the total store in the body (about twenty-five milligrams). Deficiency can develop within a few weeks on low intake and is probably the vitamin deficiency most quick to develop in people who for any reason have appetite loss.

Foods rich in the vitamin include whole-grain flours, breads and cereals, liver, lean pork, and fresh green vegetables. But the vitamin can be destroyed by overcooking and is often lost when the pot liquor of vegetables and stock from meat stews are discarded.

Riboflavin (Vitamin B_2)

For fifty-six days in 1973, a group of conscientious objectors served as volunteers in a study at the U.S. Army Medical Research and Nutrition Laboratory at Fitzsimmons General Hospital, Den-ver. They lived on an otherwise excellent diet, but one containing virtually no riboflavin.

Well before the study ended, the men began to show marked personality changes. They became increasingly depressed, hypo-chondriacal, and even verged toward hysteria. Obviously, riboflavin has effects on behavior.

The vitamin has many functions in the body, and a deficiency can produce other symptoms as well, including reduced visual acuity, eye fatigue, oversensitivity to light, seborrheic dermatitis.

One might suppose that riboflavin deficiency would be rare in the United States. Milk is a good source of it, but milk exposed to sunlight for just three and a half hours can lose as much as 75 percent of its riboflavin content. Other good sources include other dairy products and eggs, organ meats (such as liver, kidney, and heart), other meats and poultry, fish, green leafy vegetables, legumes, fruits, and nuts.

But the vitamin can be destroyed when sodium bicarbonate is used in cooking, and bread fortified with B_2 can lose some of it on exposure to light.

Niacin (B_3)

Niacin—also sometimes referred to as nicotinic acid, niacinamide, and nicotinamide—is the antipellagra vitamin. Pellagra, a nasty disease, is characterized by the four D's—dermatitis (rough skin), diarrhea, dementia, and death (if not overcome).

Niacin was discovered only about forty years ago. When it very quickly proved to be the specific cure and preventive for pellagra, a tremendous impetus was given to modern biological psychiatry, which holds that some, perhaps many, mental disturbances may have physical rather than psychological roots.

By 1955, there were reports of a variety of psychiatric disturbances that could, at least sometimes, result from niacin deficiency and that responded to treatment with the vitamin. They included some depressions, delirium, confusional exhaustion, and neurasthenia or "nervous prostration," with fatigue, appetite loss, energy deficiency, and aches and pains.

Niacin is present in many foods, including fish, organ meats, whole-grain breads and cereals, eggs, milk, poultry, lima beans, and peanuts. But deficiencies of the vitamin occur. They may result from prolonged diarrheal disease, cirrhosis of the liver, and excessive alcohol use. Simple dietary deficiency—inadequate intake of niacin-rich foods—can occur and is enough of a threat so that the Food and Nutrition Board advocates including niacin along with other nutrients that it recommends for increased fortification of foods made of wheat, corn, and rice.

Pyridoxine (Vitamin B$_6$)

First identified in 1934, pyridoxine came into the public spot-
light in 1952, when a commercial infant formula caused convulsions and the reason proved to be that excessive heating during
preparation of the formula destroyed pyridoxine. The infants
recovered quickly upon receiving the vitamin.

Not long afterward, a possible relationship between mental
retardation and increased need for pyridoxine was indicated
when retarded children suffering from convulsions were freed
of the convulsions through increased amounts of the vitamin.

Some investigators believe that there are some people who
are pyridoxine-dependent; that is, they require greater amounts
of the vitamin than normal. For example, Dr. Bernard Rimland
of the Institute for Child Behavior Research, San Diego, studied
800 psychiatric child patients and found a need for the vitamin
ranging from 5 to 400 milligrams a day although the estimated
average need in the general population is only about 3.5 milligrams.

Some men experience an anemia that produces lack of energy,
easy fatigability, and irritability, sometimes accompanied by
headache, vertigo, ear ringing, and spots before the eyes. They
seem to be pyridoxine-dependent and respond to doses of the
vitamin ranging from 50 to 200 milligrams a day.

Aside from possible special needs for large amounts of B$_6$
by people who may be dependent, is deficiency of the vitamin
common among others? There is increasing evidence that it
is. Some reports indicate that the general requirement for about
three and a half milligrams a day may be about two and a half
times as much as many people ordinarily get.

Pyridoxine is widely distributed in foods. Rich sources are
beef liver, kidney, pork loin and ham, leg of veal, fresh fish,
bananas, cabbage, avocados, peanuts, walnuts, raisins, prunes,
and cereal grains.

But vegetables lose some B_6 in freezing, and high temperatures of sterilization for canning destroy the vitamin. Cereal grains lose 80 to 90 percent of their B_6 during milling, so that commonly used flours and breads and other food products made from those flours are almost always low in the vitamin.

Cobalamin (Vitamin B_{12})

B_{12} is unique in some ways among vitamins and all compounds familiar in medicine.

It is the most complex vitamin—known to be needed for red blood cell formation and for normal nerve cell growth and maintenance. It is also suspected of having other still largely unexplored functions affecting the body in many ways.

Yet the amount required is almost incredibly small. A single microgram—one-millionth of a gram, a gram being only $\frac{1}{28}$th of an ounce—in the diet can suffice.

But B_{12} deficiency, as we noted in Chapter 6, can occur and lead to pernicious anemia, despite a good intake of the vitamin, when an intrinsic factor needed for absorption and produced by stomach cells is inadequate or lacking. And, as we noted, too, B_{12} deficiency occurs most commonly among older people.

It may be insidious in onset. Early symptoms can vary. Often, to begin with, there may be only a slight soreness of the tongue, a few mild, unalarming pins-and-needles sensations of hands or feet. At some later point, mild at first but progressively intensifying gastrointestinal symptoms may develop—appetite loss, diarrhea, episodes of nausea or abdominal pain.

The lining of the mouth may become pale, sometimes even greenish-yellow, except for the tongue, which may be bright red. The mouth may also burn, itch, or sting; and there may be discomfort upon drinking hot or cold liquids.

As deficiency persists, other symptoms may develop: weakness, shortness of breath, or palpitations (heartbeats so unusually rapid, strong, or irregular that the victim becomes very conscious of them).

At some point, nervous system symptoms develop: memory impairment, dulling of mental awareness and acuity, difficulty in concentration. There may also be disturbances of normal bladder and bowel control, persistent numbness and tingling of the extremities, and unsteadiness in walking, especially in the dark.

Provided the symptoms of B_{12} deficiency are recognized for what they are—and the earlier the better in order to avoid any possible irreversible damage to nerves—vitamin B_{12} administration can produce dramatic improvement.

Folic Acid

This B vitamin has received increasing attention recently and has become a matter of concern. Even as research has been showing its multifaceted importance, it has become apparent that deficiency of it is common.

Folic acid deficiency can lead to fatigue, headaches, constipation, sensations of dizziness, and vision blurring. In some cases, it may be responsible for weakness, irritability, sleeplessness, forgetfulness, and depression.

A deficiency can be induced readily. Body stores of the vitamin are limited, about enough to last a month. The vitamin occurs in many plant and animal tissues. Among the richest sources are yeast, liver, and green vegetables; moderate amounts are found in dairy foods, meat, and fish.

But folic acid is destroyed by heat. Cooking, especially boiling, and heat preservation in canning can destroy up to 90 percent of it. The vitamin is also unstable when exposed to air and to ultraviolet light and declines steadily in storage. So a deficiency may occur not only when leafy vegetables, fresh foods, and liver are lacking in the diet, but also when they are stored too long under bad conditions or cooked too long or overly processed.

Folic acid may be depleted, too, and supplementation with the vitamin needed when some drugs are used. They include oral contraceptives; phenobarbitone, phenytoin, and primidone, which are used for seizures; methotrexate sometimes used for cancer and severe psoriasis; and pyrimethamine, an antimalarial.

Potassium

Among the forty-odd nutrients known to be essential to man—including carbohydrates, fats, amino acids (in proteins), and vitamins—are a number of essential minerals. One of these is potassium.

Some diuretics, or "water pills," used for high blood pressure, congestive heart failure, and other conditions, in the process of promoting excretion of salt and fluids also cause a loss of potassium (called hypokalemia).

Potassium depletion may show itself in muscle weakness, cramps, diarrhea, vomiting, appetite loss, apathy, and listlessness. In severe cases, the depletion may lead to irregular heartbeat and heart muscle weakness.

Potassium depletion requires special attention to an intake of foods rich in the mineral and, in some cases, to potassium supplementation.

Potassium is widely distributed in foods, especially in meats, milk, vegetables, and fruits. Oranges, bananas, and tomatoes are especially good sources.

Magnesium

Only recently has the importance of another mineral, magnesium, begun to be recognized. It is now known to be involved in many aspects of body chemistry. It is essential for the activation of enzyme systems needed for proper use of other minerals, some vitamins, and even proteins. It is required for both nerve and muscle activity.

In recent studies, magnesium deficiency has been found capable of producing many physical disturbances, including abnormal heart rhythms, and twitching and tremors of muscles.

According to recent reports, magnesium deficiency may produce mental symptoms that can range from relatively mild apathy and memory impairment to confusion, disorientation, hallucinations, and paranoia.

At a special international conference on magnesium held at the University of Montreal not long ago, Dr. Edmund B. Flick of the West Virginia University Department of Medicine keynoted the research results presented by many investigating teams by underscoring the fact that magnesium deficiency manifestations are many and varied; that the deficiency is common; and that, although common, it often goes undetected.

When, for example, University of Colorado Hospital investigators did a special study to check on magnesium deficiency, they found it in 205, or 14.5 percent, of 1418 patients. They found, too, that commonly the physicians who were treating the patients had no suspicion that the deficiency was present and would not have requested a test for it.

Although nobody knows how widespread magnesium deficiency may be, there is concern that it may be common and growing more so. For one thing, increased softening of water may be responsible to some extent. Along with calcium, magnesium is what imparts hardness to water, and much of it is removed in the softening process.

Another significant factor could be the use of highly refined flour. Minerals as well as vitamins are lost in the heavy milling of grain, which involves the stripping away of virtually all of the mineral- and vitamin-rich bran. And when flour and bread "enrichment" programs were introduced years ago, no provision was made for enrichment with magnesium.

Some authorities now urge that when a home water softening

system is installed, at least one faucet should be left to provide untreated water. And the use of whole-grain cereals and breads could help considerably to prevent magnesium deficiency.

Zinc

Zinc is another mineral whose multiple importance has only recently become evident.

One of the first significant discoveries about zinc was that when the oral zinc supplement was tried in patients after surgery, wound healing that had previously been delayed speeded up. It appeared that after surgery—and in severe burn cases as well— even in some patients with previously adequate body stores of zinc, there might be depletion enough to interfere with healing.

Another important development came in 1971, when National Institutes of Health researchers discovered that zinc deficiency often was the cause of lost or perverted senses of taste and smell in people whose problem had previously been considered psychogenic. The researchers studied some 4000 men and women, aged twenty-five to eighty-one with taste and smell disturbances. All had low blood levels of zinc; all responded to zinc supplements.

That zinc deficiency may sometimes be responsible for mental changes—memory impairment, disorientation, depression—and that these can be overcome by zinc supplementation has been shown in recent work at the Baylor College of Medicine.

Nobody knows how common zinc deficiency may be but some authorities are convinced that it is far from rare.

One of the pioneer zinc investigators, Dr. Harold H. Sandstead of the U.S. Department of Agriculture Human Nutrition Laboratory, Grand Forks, North Dakota, observes: "The hypothesis that zinc nutriture of many Americans is marginal would have seemed ridiculous several years ago. Today, this is no longer the case. Advances in knowledge of the metabolic role of zinc, factors which influence its availability for absorption, and the effects of zinc deficiency in many have made it apparent that we must be concerned with the adequacy of the American diet as a source of zinc and with human zinc requirements."

Dr. Richard W. Luecke of Michigan State University has reported that "There is ample reason to suspect that zinc intakes of a number of individuals in this country may be marginal. Zinc shortages can be found in all people, rich or poor."

Studies have indicated that the average American diet contains eight to sixteen milligrams of zinc per day, that the average healthy person requires at least twelve milligrams daily, and that illness or injury increases the requirements.

Zinc is—or should be—widely distributed in foods. But it is largely removed from wheat and other grains and from sugar during refining. And there is some concern among Department of Agriculture experts that there is a growing zinc deficiency in plants, with deficiencies discovered in plants in at least thirty states. One troubled prediction is that unless leached-out soil zinc is replaced on a large scale, more and more people will develop symptoms of zinc deficiency.

The natural zinc content of food varies considerably. In parts of zinc per million parts of food, the averages are: seafoods, 17.5; meats, 30.6; dairy products, 8.8; cereals and grains, 17.7; legume vegetables, 10.7; root vegetables, 3.4; leafy vegetables, 1.7; fats and oils, 8.4; nuts, 34.2; fruits, 0.5; beverages, 0.2; condiments, 22.9.

Zinc content also varies within food groups. Fresh oysters, for example, contain 1487 parts per million; canned tuna, 29.1; canned sardines, 29.1; frozen shrimp, 14.8; frozen lobster, 1.5. Among meats, round steak with 56.6 and lamb chops with 55.3 are richest; ground beef contains 25 parts per million; liver, 39.2; pork loin, 18.9; pork chops, 3.6; chicken legs, 29.1. Whole egg contains 20.8; nonfat dry milk, 35.1; homogenized milk, only 0.5 or less. Among condiments, caraway seeds contain 2.8; cinnamon, 13.4; black pepper, 18.3; and ground mustard, 22.9.

WHAT DO OLDER PEOPLE REALLY NEED?

Except under unusual circumstances, older people need less total quantity but the same types of foods that, ideally, younger people should have.

It is a fact that there is an increased incidence of obesity among the elderly, and two major factors account for it.

One is that the basal metabolic rate—the rate at which the body utilizes energy—decreases with age. After early adulthood, the rate falls by about 2 percent each decade.

The more important factor leading to obesity is decreased physical activity. Although it is difficult to determine the actual decrease in physical activity with age, one authoritative estimate is that activity patterns decrease by about 200 kilocalories a day in men between the ages of forty-five and seventy-five and by about 500 kilocalories a day after age seventy-five compared to men between the ages of twenty and forty-five.

To offset the reduced basal metabolic rate and decreased physical activity, the National Research Council recommends a reduction to 90 percent of energy allowances needed by people fifty years and older. This means a decrease of 200 to 300 calories, or an intake of about 2400 calories for men and 1800 for women over fifty.

But if there is need for fewer calories with aging, it is still a fact that older people need almost the same amount of essential nutrients as younger adults. The requirements for protein, minerals, vitamins, and other essentials are not less; but with less total food intake, the density of nutrients should be greater.

That means far less room in the diet of an older person for "empty calories"—for such items as candy and soft drinks.

Four basic food groups should provide the basis for an older person's dietary regimen. Those sources of nutrients are:

1. Meat and allied foods: meat, poultry, eggs, and fish. These supply protein, fat, iron, and vitamins.

2. Dairy products: whole, skimmed, evaporated, or dried milk, and milk products such as cheese, butter, and buttermilk. These supply calcium, proteins, fat, and vitamins.

3. Vegetables and fruits. These supply vitamins, minerals, and fiber. It is important to include citrus fruit for vitamin C and dark green or yellow vegetables or fruit for vitamin A.

4. Bread and cereals. These provide proteins, iron, and B vitamins as well as carbohydrates. Enriched flour and cornmeal offer vitamins B_1 and B_2, niacin, and iron. And whole-grain flour, bread, and brown rice contain other B vitamins, minerals, and desirable fiber.

During preparation of foods one should avoid unnecessary use of fats, gravies, and sugars.

Within each food group, lower calorie foods should be given preference—for example, skim milk instead of whole milk, and fish, chicken, or eggs instead of pork or beef.

Balance—Plus Variety

With foods each day from the four groups, a diet will be balanced.

No less important may be varying choices within each group.

Every physician and scientist concerned with nutrition knows well that despite all that has been learned, nutrition is a young science and much more remains to be learned. Knowledge about many vitamins, for example, dates back only a few decades. And recognition of the importance of some minerals is even more recent.

At any time, some fundamental new finding—of a previously unknown vitamin or other essential nutrient—may be made. Nature distributes her largesse. We can be most certain of benefiting from it by making use of many rather than limited numbers of food items. Almost certainly if we do this, we will be enjoying the values of still-undiscovered vital elements.

A Note About Fiber

Only very recently has come the discovery that something which in recent times has been largely missing from the American diet may be related to a wide variety of health problems.

The missing ingredient, dietary fiber—sometimes called bulk or roughage—hardly seems capable at first blush of being of great importance.

Until recent times, man ate much fiber. It's the indigestible part of plant cell walls, present in large amounts in grains and cereals.

But about the turn of the century, the invention of modern roller mills made it possible economically to remove the outer husk of cereal grain kernels, and with it the fiber, to produce refined white flour.

Ever since, fiber intake has plummeted. Today, cereal fiber intake in the United States is one-tenth of what it was.

And even as fiber intake has decreased, the incidence of many diseases has increased. Appendicitis, for example, became common only in this century, hiatus hernia only in the last thirty years; coronary heart disease was considered a rarity fifty years ago.

Yet nothing comparable has occurred among rural Africans living on native unrefined diets. They get infections; they sometimes go hungry; but eating unrefined cereal as a staple, getting about twenty-five grams of fiber a day—many times as much as the average American—they rarely experience the chronic Western diseases.

Why is fiber important?

Fibrous foods add bulk. In the intestinal tract the fiber absorbs water. That makes stools soft and large. And that prevents constipation, with its small, hard, pebbly, slow-moving stools. Typically, native African stools weigh up to four times those of Westerners; and transit time—the time it takes food to pass through the body—averages only thirty-five hours for Africans but ninety hours for many Westerners.

Constipation—rare in rural Africans—leads to straining. Straining raises pressure in the colon, which pushes on the colon wall, causing the outpouching of diverticular disease, a common painful problem in people beyond forty. Intra-abdominal pressure also is raised and may push the stomach up through the diaphragm, producing hiatus hernia, with its heartburn, regurgitation of stomach acid back up into the esophagus, and burning pain in back of the breastbone.

Raised pressure in the abdomen also can be transmitted elsewhere—to the leg veins, dilating them so they become varicose veins, and to veins in the anal region, causing hemorrhoids.

Cancer of the colon is believed to result from carcinogens (cancer-producing chemicals) made by bacteria in the bowel. With small, hard, constipated, slow-moving stools, the bacteria have more time to act; and the carcinogens they produce are more concentrated in the small stools and also are retained and can act for longer periods on the lining of the colon.

Coronary heart disease, forerunner of heart attacks, may be related at least in part to lack of fiber in the diet. Many studies indicate that people on high-fiber diets have lower blood cholesterol levels and less cholesterol deposits in the coronary arteries feeding the heart.

Evidence that restoring fiber to the diet can achieve some remarkable effects is accumulating.

In a study with adults and children, the substitution of just two slices of fiber-rich whole meal bread for the same amount of white bread and the addition of two teaspoonsful of fiber-rich bran a day led, within three weeks, to marked increases in stool weight and speed-up of transit time, with an end to constipation. Many hemorrhoid sufferers have been relieved as stools have softened.

Until just half a dozen years ago, roughage was banned for people with diverticular disease. Now physicians report that adding fiber to the diet produces real benefits. In one large study, 88.6 percent of patients improved, and many who had been scheduled for surgery no longer required it.

The irritable bowel syndrome—also called spastic colon and mucous colitis—is a problem in more than half of patients seeking medical help for gastrointestinal troubles without organic abnormalities. They may suffer chronically from abdominal distention, cramps, or dull deep pain, and sometimes heartburn, excessive belching, nausea, weakness, and headaches. Irritable colon has responded gratifying to a high-fiber diet in several studies.

Long-term investigation of what dietary fiber may do for other problems, including diabetes and heart disease, is under way.

Meanwhile, there is evidence of fiber's value in combating obesity.

Providing no calories, it takes the place of other foods that do. Fiber also requires chewing, which slows intake and also limits it by increasing the secretion of both saliva and gastric juice that serve to distend the stomach and help produce satiety.

Moreover, fiber cuts down on body absorption of other foods. Investigators have determined that where 97 percent of total dietary energy is absorbed on a low-fiber diet, only 92.5 percent is absorbed on a high-fiber diet.

At Britain's University of Bristol, Dr. Kenneth Heaton, doing pioneering studies on fiber and obesity, has noted losses of ten, fifteen, and more pounds in volunteers—including himself and his wife, also a physician—who simply restored fiber to their diets without paying any special attention to calories.

How do you put fiber back in your diet?

You can do it in several ways. You can use oatmeal (the old-fashioned slow-cooking kind, not "instant"), whole grain wheat cereal designed to be cooked, or shredded wheat. And you can now find commercial whole meal breads and whole meal flour that can be used at home to make bread, rolls, muffins, and pancakes.

Seeds—such as whole sesame and sunflower—along with seed-filled berries, such as raspberries, blackberries, and loganberries, provide fiber.

So do many fruits and vegetables, raw or only lightly cooked. (Cooking tends to break down fiber, and the more cooking, the more breakdown.)

A study of more than twenty fruits and vegetables indicates them to be valuable for fiber content in this order: mango, carrot, apple, brussels sprout, eggplant, spring cabbage, orange, pear, green bean, lettuce, winter cabbage, pea, onion, celery, cucumber, broad bean, tomato, cauliflower, banana, rhubarb, old potato, new potato, turnip. As much as possible, fruit skins should be eaten for their fiber content.

You can also use bran, a material removed when flour is milled. It's available in breakfast cereals with "bran" in their names and also as unprocessed bran available in health food stores and many supermarkets. You can sprinkle unprocessed bran on cereals or mix it with soup or with flour in baking.

Guidelines on Conserving Nutrients

Vegetables and fruits. Wash quickly without soaking. Minimize peeling; cook whole, with skins on, whenever possible. Peeling and slicing cause as much as a 50 percent loss of vitamin C.

Avoid thawing frozen vegetables and fruits until immediately before cooking, or they lose nutrients. Store fresh fruits and vegetables only briefly before preparing and serving.

Don't drain liquid from canned vegetables; it contains 40 percent of the vitamin C, as much as a third of the B_1 and B_2. Cook with it and save what is left for soups and sauces. Note, too, that as much as half the vitamins in a can of fruit are in the liquid.

Trim very skimpily such leafy vegetables as lettuce and cabbage; nutrient concentration is greater in the outer rather than inner leaves.

Don't overcook frozen vegetables—they are already par-boiled—and just heat and serve canned goods.

Drop fruits and vegetables into already boiling water (at high temperature, because of the effect of an enzyme system in the foods, there is less destruction of vitamin C), cover, bring to boil again, and cook only until firm and tender. Better yet, use a steamer so vegetables don't soak in water.

Do not use baking soda in cooking yellow or green vegetables; it destroys vitamin B_1.

Meats. The higher the temperature in cooking, the greater the shrinking and drying—and also the loss of nutrients. Cook at moderate temperatures—300 to 350 degrees—and avoid over-cooking. That includes pork, which, because of the risk of trichinosis, many people "cook to death." Trichinae are destroyed at 140 degrees, and pork cooked at 325 degrees for thirty minutes a pound is safe—and also more nutritious.

Roasting and broiling are the best ways of cooking meat from the standpoint of nutrient retention. In broiling, too, much of the fat drips off and can be discarded. Frying may actually double the calorie count.

Fish and shellfish. Broil or bake fish at 400 degrees, leaving on the skin (and even head and tail until you serve, if you are cooking a whole fish) to prevent loss of juices and nutrients.

Steam lobsters and crabs in their shells to help preserve nutrient content. An exception is shrimp, which can be shelled, since cooking time is only three to five minutes, minimizing nutrient loss.

Cereals and pasta. Simmer rice, barley, and other cereals in no more than about twice as much water as cereal. Cook pasta in already boiling water, drain, and serve.

12

And Still Other Correctables

When a seventy-three-year-old woman falls while waiting for a bus, many people are apt to attribute it to senility. However, Dr. Harold L. Klawans of the Division of Neurology at Michael Reese Medical Center, Chicago, became suspicious of possible medical causes when several elderly people came to him with the same complaint of unexplained falling.

Klawans and his colleague Dr. Jordan L. Topel of Rush-Presbyterian–St. Luke's Medical Center, Chicago, examined eleven such patients, who were sixty-four years of age or older. Each was given a thorough physical check, plus six tests of their nervous systems. All failed the one for postural reflexes.

The test seems crude to the uninitiated. The physician gives a sudden push to the patient's chest. When postural reflexes are normal, the patient maintains balance, usually with a short backward step. But the postural reflexes of these elderly people were so impaired that they would have fallen backward from the push had not someone been there to catch them.

Further examination led the two physicians to conclude that these patients had the neurological condition known as parkinsonism, or shaking palsy. None had been so diagnosed previously, probably because they did not have any of the usual par-

162

kinsonism signs: stooped, shuffling gait; shaking of the hands; "pill-rolling" motion of the fingers.

Happily, Klawans and Topel could report in the *Journal of the American Medical Association,* the "falling sickness" was alleviated in all eleven patients with either of two medicines—L-dopa or amantadine—which have helped thousands of parkinsonism patients.

Klawans and Topel had shown that alertness and a high degree of suspicion that all is not senility can be rewarding.

That was equally true in the case of an elderly widow who was transferred to the Vanderbilt University Hospital in Nashville after hospitalization elsewhere because of periods of psychotic excitement that alternated with periods of clouded consciousness.

Her health had been excellent until six years before, when she had developed the signs and symptoms of hypothyroidism. Since then she had needed daily thyroid treatment to make up for the inadequate thyroid gland functioning. A year before, her husband had died and she had handled that well.

Five months before hospital admission, she had a dizzy spell and briefly lost consciousness. No cause for this was established. Several months later, the patient abruptly developed insomnia, early morning awakening, severe depression, nightmares, and auditory hallucinations. At that point, she had been admitted to the local hospital appearing deeply depressed, but her symptoms cleared quickly without specific treatment.

A week later, however, her behavior became unusual. Again she was admitted to the local hospital, but her thinking improved spontaneously within a few hours and she appeared to be herself again. Three days later, she became withdrawn, refused to eat, and thereafter became restless, fitful, and irritable and experienced bouts of violent anger that required restraints.

On arrival at Vanderbilt University Hospital, she was hostile, agitated at times to the point of needing restraints, at other times rigid. She assumed bizarre postures, reported hearing voices, her speech became disorganized.

At Vanderbilt, physicians became suspicious, carried out brain wave (electroencephalographic) studies, found abnormalities. Upon receiving anticonvulsant medication, she recovered promptly, described her experience as much like that of recovering from a bad dream. She was discharged on a regimen of anticonvulsant medication and has remained well.

She had been a victim not of senility or of true psychosis. Instead, she had suffered from what is called transient ictal psychosis—a condition in which psychotic episodes appear in conjunction with epilepticlike brain wave patterns often in the absence of apparent epileptic seizures.

The two cases help to illustrate a fact, already noted throughout much of this book, that much of what can appear to be hopeless mental deterioration in an older person is not hopeless at all.

Many physical problems, if long endured without relief and without hope, can contribute to mental decline in older people; and yet many of these problems are not hopeless.

The nature of some of them is obvious; and yet too often, particularly when it comes to older victims, they are approached with a feeling of needless defeatism, sometimes by the victims but sometimes, too, by physicians. Some are not so obvious in nature.

The "Great Imposter"

When he turned up in the office of a New York City dentist, the man with chronic head pain that had bothered him for years and grown progressively worse was desperate. He had made a round of physicians. He had sought help unsuccessfully, he explained, from an internist, a neurologist, a nose and throat specialist, and an orthopedic surgeon.

"How," the dentist wondered, "did you miss seeing a psychiatrist?"

"I'm a psychiatrist myself," the patient announced, "and this is not psychosomatic pain."

It wasn't. Quickly, the dentist could pinpoint and effectively treat the problem: TMJ (temporomandibular joint) dysfunction—a lower jaw problem.

The TMJ condition, which has been nicknamed the "Great Imposter" because it can produce a wide variety of symptoms and mimic many different diseases, is estimated to affect 20 percent of the population to some degree—and is completely overlooked in most.

Victims of TMJ dysfunction, reports Dr. Douglas H. Morgan of White Memorial Medical Center, Los Angeles, "are the persons who go from doctor to doctor with a multitude of seemingly unrelated symptoms. In some, there may be functional problems—an inability to open or close the mouth. In others, there may be only pain that resembles migraine, sinus problems, atypical facial pain mimicking a tic douloureux or a temporal arteritis, or neck and shoulder pain. In others, there may be no pain, only dizziness, tinnitus [ear ringing], or subjective hearing loss."

Says Dr. Nathan A. Shore, lecturer at the New York University College of Dentistry, who has treated more than 2800 TMJ patients: "Many have been told they are psychosomatically ill and must learn to live with their 'imaginary' pains. The fact is that it's the pain that makes them neurotic, not neurosis that causes the pain."

The temporomandibular joint is in front of the ear, where the lower jaw (or mandible) hinges to the skull. The joint can get out of adjustment from a blow to head or jaw, or from opening the jaw too wide or too long during biting or yawning. A poor bite can cause trouble. So can clenching or gnashing the teeth under tension or stress.

Once the joint is affected, the equilibrium of muscles and ligaments controlling joint movement is upset. In response, the muscles go into spasm, or involuntary contraction, a painful state.

And the pain then may radiate a considerable distance, shooting out from small areas of great sensitivity—called trigger points—within muscles. Trigger points in the TMJ muscle system can produce dull ache or stabbing pain not only around jaw and teeth but virtually anywhere in the head, neck, and shoulders.

Yet, if the possibility of TMJ dysfunction is considered, accurate diagnosis need not be difficult.

Patients themselves may have reason to suspect it when jaw or other pain is relieved with opening of the mouth but is intensified on chewing, speaking, and brushing the teeth; when the jaws are found to be clenched upon awakening; or when there is awareness of tooth grinding during moments of concentration.

To help in diagnosis, Dr. Shore has developed simple tests which, he reports, can be carried out in a minute by any physician or dentist.

One involves simply listening by ear or with a stethoscope for any clicking or crepitous noises (similar to those of walking on gravel) when the jaw is moved. Another is to see if the jaw waves from side to side when the mouth is opened.

Others include feeling (palpating) the temporomandibular joint on each side, and the muscles as well, to detect any spasm.

In many hundreds of patients, Dr. Shore reports, a temporary plastic appliance—a removable biteplate—that is fitted to the upper teeth has been used successfully. By keeping the upper teeth separated from the lower, it helps the lower jaw move into proper position and overcomes spasm, so the joint gradually resumes normal function. The biteplate is worn almost constantly, except for eating and tooth brushing, for about four months.

In some cases, it's necessary to restore balance in use of jaw muscles. Many people tend to use only one side of the mouth during chewing. In addition to making a conscious effort to chew on the other side as well, they may be asked to perform simple exercises. In one, the tip of the tongue is placed far back on the roof of the mouth and the mouth is then opened wide; this helps balance the jaw muscles and control crackling. In another, the jaw is moved a given number of times away from the weak side to strengthen the muscles.

To combat spasm, patients may be asked to apply moist heat for ten minutes three times a day to both sides of the face and eat soft foods for a time.

The results can be impressive.

One study at the TMJ clinics of the French and Polyclinic Medical School and the New York Eye and Ear Infirmary included 112 patients with chronic headaches who had been referred after unsuccessful treatment from a headache clinic, all of whom proved to be TMJ victims. With treatment, headaches improved in all but nine, with sixty-five becoming entirely free of them. Of sixteen who had also suffered from vertigo, twelve were helped; of twenty with ear pain, nineteen benefited; and of thirty-eight with ear noises, all but seven were helped.

In a study at the University of North Carolina Dental School, Chapel Hill, by Dr. Ernest W. Small, forty-three of fifty patients with deep pain in the side of the face got relief from TMJ treatment.

Recently, many hospitals and dental schools have set up special clinics for TMJ dysfunction. A team approach is often used—with a dentist, ear-nose-and-throat specialist, neurologist, and other specialists working together.

And the importance of the TMJ problem is finally beginning to be recognized by a broader segment of the medical and dental professions.

"There is gradually developing," says Dr. Morgan of White Memorial, "a group of dentists and physicians interested and knowledgeable in this area. More TMJ clinics will be developed in dental schools and hospitals. Roentgenographic [x-ray] techniques involving the joint are being improved and refined. The future holds more hope for the large numbers afflicted with this severe and perplexing problem."

Arthritis

"It's such a wonderful feeling to walk once again to the podium without pain or embarrassment. It's like getting a whole new lease on life." With those words, then seventy-three-year-old Eugene Ormandy, director of the Philadelphia Orchestra, summed up what one advance in surgical treatment of crippling arthritis had meant to him.

Before undergoing surgery at the age of seventy-two, Mr. Ormandy walked with a pronounced limp and great pain because of osteoarthritis of his left hip. Within weeks after his hip joint was replaced with an artificial joint, he could walk normally, go up and down stairs, without the slightest pain or trace of a limp.

It has been said that if most people consider a diagnosis of cancer to be a sentence of death, they look upon arthritis as a sentence of life imprisonment. Neither is necessarily true.

Arthritis today often can be helped. Surgery can work wonders in many cases when medical measures prove inadequate. And it is also true that medical measures, when properly used by a knowledgeable physician, can be of great value.

A major problem has been that arthritis has not been, and still is not, curable, even though it is often controllable. And many people—many physicians among them—are cure-oriented.

Writing recently on "Rehabilitation of the Elderly," Dr. T. E. Hunt, professor of rehabilitation and geriatric medicine at the University of Saskatchewan, Saskatoon, Canada, reported: "I recall an elderly woman whose arthritis was untreated for 30 years. Her physician, a general practitioner, did nothing for her because 'you can't cure arthritis.' She was never referred to a rehabilitation or rheumatic disease unit where the disease might have been controlled and where she certainly would have achieved greater functional independence. This was not misdiagnosis but mismanagement—nihilism engendered by the physician's orientation toward 'cure.'

"Of course," Dr. Hunt also observed, "the reverse attitude often prevails as well—that is that the restorative potential is assumed to be nonexistent or much less than is actually the case because the patient is old. In the past many elderly disabled have been denied perfectly feasible rehabilitation services because of their advanced age."

Rheumatoid arthritis. Of the types of arthritis which are most widespread, affecting at least 20 million Americans who suffer from the most severe forms and 20 million others to milder degree, rheumatoid arthritis is the most serious, painful, and potentially crippling.

A systemic illness, rheumatoid arthritis often begins with nonspecific symptoms such as fever, chills, poor appetite, and a general rundown feeling. Later, joints become inflamed, stiff, sore, and painful. Most often, the joints of fingers, wrists, knees, ankles, and toes, alone or in combination, are affected, although all joints may be involved.

In one type of rheumatoid arthritis, there is severe joint inflammation, with pain, swelling, and fairly rapidly developing deformities. Fever and prostration often accompany this type, and if the disease is not treated, crippling deformities may soon occur. More commonly, the pain and swelling are not as severe and disabling at first, and there may be intervals during which few if any symptoms are experienced. Gradually, however, over many years and often after several attacks of more severe joint pain, the joints may become deformed.

Because the cause of rheumatoid arthritis still is not known, there are no basic means of prevention. But measures to treat the disease are available.

Aspirin is the mainstay of treatment, yet an often misunderstood one. As an expert committee of the American Rheumatism

Association has pointed out, aspirin must be taken in adequate amounts if it is to have any value. Beyond its ability to relieve pain and fever, the drug has an anti-inflammatory action but only in higher dosages. It's this anti-inflammatory effect which is important in rheumatoid arthritis. Upwards of eight tablets a day may be required on a regular basis. Not all patients tolerate this amount of aspirin well, but many do and benefit.

Periods of rest during the day are helpful, but complete inactivity is to be avoided unless there is severe disease with markedly painful, swollen joints. Heat is an excellent means of obtaining temporary relief—dry heat through electric pads and hot water bottles and wet heat through fifteen-minute hot baths and wet packs.

Other drugs such as indomethacin and antimalarials are sometimes effective when aspirin is not adequate. Gold salt treatment is often valuable. Usually a patient receives a test injection of a small amount of gold, and if there are no undesirable reactions, this is followed by weekly injections of fifty milligrams. Improvement seldom occurs until 200 to 400 milligrams have been given. If no change occurs after administration of a full gram, 1000 milligrams, the injections may be stopped. But if, as often happens, there is significant improvement, the patient may then continue to receive maintenance injections at about monthly intervals.

Under the expert care of a rheumatologist, rheumatoid arthritis, although it cannot be cured, very often can be made to go into remission. Such care may require the use of every available approach.

Effective treatment, as Dr. James S. Paolino of St. Vincent's Hospital and Medical Center, New York City, has pointed out, "does not imply passive observation, but rather the vigorous employment of all current modalities, rationally selected. The result can be highly rewarding."

One example of this is an elderly woman whose rheumatoid arthritis began with what seemed to be recurrent "bursitis" of both shoulders, which was treated intermittently with aspirin, codeine, and local heat, providing enough relief so she could continue to be active.

A year later, aching, stiffness, and swelling affected her hands and wrists. She found relief by soaking her hands in warm water for fifteen minutes each morning and by intermittent use of warm paraffin, long hot baths, and short courses of a drug, phenylbutazone. Then four years later, the pain in her hands became more severe and prolonged, and pain and swelling affected a foot.

Finally she was fitted with an ankle brace and started on gold therapy. After ten weekly injections of gold, her foot swelling began to subside. After another three injections, she was free of all symptoms. Two years later, with at most two aspirins in the morning followed by a hot bath and use of the foot brace, she is pain-free and functional all day long.

Osteoarthritis. Also known as degenerative joint disease, osteoarthritis does not usually develop before middle age except when a joint has been injured or when joints have been subjected to much stress and overuse, as in the fingers of some pianists.

Ordinarily, it is a mildly uncomfortable disease. Unlike rheumatoid arthritis, it produces no constitutional symptoms such as fever. In some cases, however, it may cause joint disability. The joints most often affected are the weight-bearing ones such as hips, knees, and ankles. Affected joints may "creak" and grate on movement.

The main objectives of treatment include pain relief, restoration of joint function, and prevention of avoidable disability and disease progression.

Daily periods of rest can be useful. When weight-bearing joints are affected, local support, including use of cane, crutch, or mechanical device, can be helpful. Wearing of suitable shoes, restoration of arch, or building up of one side of a shoe to shift the line of weight-bearing may be useful. So, too, weight reduction and correction of abnormal posture.

Useful local measures include heat and specific exercises designed to avoid or correct muscle wasting, since muscle weakness intensifies joint instability and contributes to disability. Here again, aspirin is useful in moderate doses.

And here again, vigorous treatment can be used effectively in many cases when osteoarthritis does not respond.

For example, finally, after three years of pain, particularly in her right hip and knee but also in both hands and right wrist, a seventy-five-year-old woman was admitted to St. Vincent's Hospital in New York. When drug therapy alone failed to bring improvement, for sixteen days she received daily treatment of both knees and hips with physical therapy, including active and passive range-of-motion exercises. Her hands were treated with paraffin and increasingly active exercise. At the time of discharge she could walk without pain with the help of a crutch, the range of motion in her right hip was significantly increased. And, taught how to use paraffin for her hands and range-of-motion exercises for her hips at home, she has since done well.

Surgery. The operating room has been called a new frontier in arthritis. The number of surgical procedures for treatment of severe, otherwise unyielding arthritis has increased tenfold over the last decade, and the curve is still rising.

It is the most severely crippled—those unable to walk or move freely, to hold a job or do normal housework—for whom surgery offers most hope, thanks to remarkable advances in developing materials compatible with the human body, greatly improved methods of adhering them, and the growth of the new field of bioengineering in which engineers and other specialists work alongside physicians to design increasingly sophisticated prosthetic devices.

One of the most dramatic developments has been total hip replacement. In the past, many efforts to devise an artificial hip had ended in failure. The material had to be strong enough to withstand the millions of loading pounds placed on the hip over a period of years, compatible with and uncorroded by body fluids and tissues, and self-lubricating. Surgeons had tried using a stainless steel ball as a replacement for the diseased femur (thigh) bone head, screwing the ball into the bone, but sometimes it came loose. They had made a socket of steel in which the ball could rotate, but a steel-to-steel joint had to be lubricated by body fluids and often these were inadequate.

Then, Dr. John Charnley, a British surgeon, decided to try the suggestion of a dentist friend that methyl methacrylate, a cement used in dentistry, might hold both ball and socket in place securely—and, for the socket, Charnley tried a plastic high-density polyethylene instead of steel.

The results—in hundreds of patients—were gratifying. Some of the patients put on dramatic demonstrations at American medical meetings. A woman, previously totally incapacitated, walked without pain or limp after both hips had been replaced. A man handicapped for more than twenty years did a "go-go" dance.

Many thousands of Americans now are walking around with man-made hip joints. Those helped include Margaret Chase Smith, former U.S. Senator from Maine, and, as mentioned previously, the conductor Eugene Ormandy.

From the beginning, American reports have been enthusiastic. At Massachusetts General Hospital, Boston, after performing more than 800 hip replacements, a team headed by Dr. Roderick E. Turner could report that 96 percent of patients gained better motion and freedom from discomfort. "The dramatic relief of pain invariably surprises the patients, most of whom can barely recall the last time they enjoyed a night of undisturbed sleep," noted Dr. Turner.

At the Mayo Clinic, after reviewing results in the first 333 hip replacement patients, followed for one to two years, Dr. Mark Coventry could report that arthritics undergoing the operation have these prospects:

- 96 percent will have no pain or only slight pain;
- 97 percent will have no limp or only slight limp;
- 93 percent will be able to climb stairs with banisters;

- 91 percent will need no support or only occasional support from a cane;
- 98 percent will be able to sit normally;
- 97 percent will be able to use public transport;
- 98 percent will have no deformity.

Are older people good candidates for the operation? Indeed. In fact, to begin with, people over fifty were the only ones most surgeons operated on, until the age limit was lowered more recently after more than a decade of experience showed that the hip replacement was long-lasting and therefore as practical for younger as for older patients.

Other crippled joints as well are now being replaced increasingly.

Total knee joint replacement has become feasible—a blessing, since the knee, bearing virtually all the body's weight, is very susceptible to arthritis and is probably the most frequently affected joint. Usually, medical treatment is helpful, but in about 10 percent of cases it fails.

A new ankle joint developed by Dr. Theodore Waugh at the University of California at Irvine can be implanted in less than an hour and provides both side-to-side and up-and-down foot motion. Most patients are up and walking on crutches in less than a week and walking unaided within a month. Some of the first to receive the new ankle joint, previously unable for years to walk without crutches, reportedly are playing golf.

Toe implants have become practical. In some cases of very severe arthritis the foot becomes deformed to the point that, for pain relief, one of the joints of the great toe must be surgically removed. But the toe then loses function and begins to drift to the side, producing new deformity and difficulty in walking. To help in such cases, a variety of prosthetic implants, including half-joints, spacers, and hinged devices have been developed. At the University of California, Los Angeles Medical Center, of the first nineteen patients to receive implants—the majority middle-aged and elderly women—most have experienced pain relief and improved toe alignment. Ten have become able to walk without limitation, and five others can walk up to six blocks at a time, Dr. Andrea Cracchiolo III has reported.

Finger joints are also in increasing use as replacements when arthritis produces severe hand deformities. And recently, prosthetic knuckles have been developed to help patients with arthritis-deformed hands no longer able to grip and pinch or to open widely enough to grasp large objects.

And still other joints—including a new shoulder joint and a promising new elbow—are coming into use.

Surgery will never be the final answer to arthritis. That will come when the origins of the arthritis diseases are known and prevention becomes possible. But arthritics need all the help they can get right now. And today, when medical therapy is not enough, surgery has much to offer.

No surgery can be considered minor. Always, there is at least a slight element of risk, some immediate discomfort. There is expense—and for a hip or knee replacement operation, for example, the bill may come to $5000 or more. In many cases, much or all of the cost may be met by medical insurance, Medicare, or Medicaid.

When surgery relieves chronic pain, restores the function of a joint, improves appearance, enables an elderly patient to be self-sufficient and lead a near normal life, its value is beyond calculation. Not least of all, it may contribute to a resurgence of spirit and mentation.

Emphysema: Help for Lung Cripples

He is now in his late sixties. For nineteen years, until not long ago, he needed hospitalization every two months. A victim of emphysema, he had had to strain for every breath and periodically was overwhelmed by attacks of such severe respiratory failure that he needed emergency treatment.

He no longer needs emergency treatment. He swims the length

of a pool seventy times a day every day of the week, plays eighteen holes of golf three times a week, walks whenever he can, operates a ham radio which he built himself, and has added bicycle riding to his daily agenda. "I feel in better shape today," he says, "than I felt in my life, although I know I am not."

And, literally speaking, he is not. But he demonstrates the validity of a relatively new concept: that emphysema victims, too long consigned to a vegetating existence, their disease written off as inevitably progressive and untreatable, deserve and can have far brighter prospects. Although they may never be brought back entirely to normal after the disease has become far advanced, they can be helped to make maximum use of their lung reserve and to lead more hopeful, active, and productive lives.

Emphysema ranks as one of our most devastating and explosive afflictions. According to the U.S. Public Health Service, it disables one of every fourteen wage earners over the age of forty-five and in recent years almost half a million new victims yearly have come under medical care. But the outlook for them has seemed grim.

The word emphysema comes from the Greek for inflation or swelling. It's descriptive of the disease in which the lungs lose their elasticity and become puffed up with air which the patient cannot expel completely. Because of the accumulation of stale air, it becomes difficult to breathe in normal amounts of fresh air. Shortness of breath develops.

Mucus in the air passages adds to the problem. In healthy people, inhaled air easily passes beyond the normally present mucus, and during exhalation, expelled air tends to push any accumulations upward so that a cough can remove them readily. In the emphysemic, however, the force of exhalation is much diminished. Mucus accumulates, becomes thick and tenacious, blocks some of the airways, adds to shortness of breath. The retained mucus also encourages bacterial growth and frequent infections.

As emphysema progresses, the patient tries to avoid any physical activity that makes him breathe hard. As activity decreases, muscles weaken, use oxygen less efficiently, and require more and more of it to do less and less work. A vicious cycle is set up.

The problem has seemed overwhelming. Commonly, the lot of the emphysema patient has been repeated emergency hospitalizations for severe attacks of respiratory failure.

Yet, given aggressive treatment, emphysema is not hopeless.

Drugs can be used to loosen and thin secretions, helping to keep the airways open. Colds and minor respiratory infections may be treated vigorously to try to avoid serious lung infection.

In some cases, periodic treatment with machines that push air into the lungs (intermittent positive-pressure breathing, or IPPB) to help open collapsed areas in order to drain mucus collections or prevent their formation may be valuable.

Exercises may be prescribed to help develop muscles ordinarily not used for breathing so as to increase breathing effectiveness.

For extreme emphysema, with breathing difficulty even while eating, talking, or at rest, lung drainage may be helpful. A tube is introduced into the trachea, or windpipe, through the mouth and a special suction tube is inserted through the first tube to remove obstructing secretions.

Some patients have benefited from a few such drainage procedures and then have required no more for extended periods but others are not helped unless lung drainage is done daily.

For the latter, now, self-drainage can be made possible by an operative procedure, tracheal fenestration, which creates an entrance to the trachea through an opening in the neck just above the breastbone. The opening, which is skin-lined, airtight, and leakproof, and does not interfere with speech, allows a patient himself to insert the tubes. Drs. M. C. Gluck and E. E. Rockey of New York Medical College have reported their experience with a group of patients who, within days to weeks after tracheal fenestration, were able to carry out their own drainage and experience significant improvement, to the point of returning to work or other activity.

A major development. In most general hospitals, emphysemics obtain excellent crisis care. They are far more likely to be discharged alive than a decade ago thanks to sophisticated emergency techniques. But commonly they require readmission weeks or months later.

A major recent development has been the establishment of special outpatient programs for emphysema patients. They may differ in detail but have much in common. They are designed to give patients sustained personal attention such as they rarely if ever have had before, to replace feelings of despair with hope, and to demonstrate to them how they can help themselves.

Among the pioneers have been the New York University Institute of Rehabilitation; Gompers Rehabilitation Center in Phoenix; Ralph K. Davies Medical Center in San Francisco; Mountaineer Breathing Clinic in Beckley, West Virginia; Gunderson Clinic in LaCrosse, Wisconsin; the Rehabilitation Institute of Chicago; the Albert Steiner Memorial Emphysema Clinic at St. Joseph's Infirmary in Atlanta; and the Velda Rose Outpatient Respiratory Care Program in Mesa, Arizona.

As an example, at the nonprofit Velda Rose Program, which was established by Dr. Fred A. Obley, a general practitioner, each month a class of a dozen or more patients is formed. The patients are referred by their physicians. Each is thoroughly examined. Over a four-week period, patients—and spouses—attend eight one-hour lectures and eight one-hour physical therapy training sessions.

They are taught lung anatomy and a variety of fundamental aids: how to use pursed-lip breathing to help keep airways open; how to rid the lungs of secretions by coughing with the aid of muscles of the diaphragm (replacing the usual shallow cough which does little more than clear the throat). They are taught postural drainage (tilting the body to help clear secretions), and

spouses are shown how to percuss or tap chest, sides, and back
to help loosen secretions.

They are given breathing exercises for use at home and each
patient is put on an individually graded and progressive program
of exercises and physical activities—walking increasingly longer
distances, or swimming more and more pool lengths (often particularly useful for patients who also have severe arthritis), or
bicycling.

To become active can be no easy matter for someone who
for years may have avoided almost all activity and who at first
may gasp at the slightest exertion. But therapists encourage;
there is also a group therapy effect; and motivation is also stimulated by round-table sessions with patients from previous classes
who can demonstrate the valuable results of the effort.

As one patient summed up the emphysema problem and what
has to be done about it: "Perhaps more than any other disease,
emphysema is one you can't sit and lick your wounds about.
It's easy to do that. You get a picture of yourself as a repulsive,
gasping, sickly-looking person from whom other people shrink.
You get a feeling from physicians, although they may never come
right out and say so, that you are doomed, must become progressively worse. You become depressed and irritable, have feelings of guilt about what you are inflicting on your family, and
retire more and more into yourself. But all of that is self-defeating. You have to face emphysema, look it in the eye, and fight
it. That's what you learn to do here."

One of those who learned to do it was the man mentioned
at the beginning of this section. According to records of the
Velda Rose Program, of the first 250 patients to participate,
more than 95 percent have experienced an improved sense of
well-being. Eighty-three percent have shown significantly increased physical capacity and endurance. Patients previously unable to walk more than a few steps without gasping have become
able in many cases to walk several miles.

Outpatient programs elsewhere are achieving comparable results. Hopefully, more and more of them will be established.

"I see no reason," says Dr. Obley, "why there shouldn't be a network of such programs across the country, making rehabilitation available to every emphysema patient. Because rehabilitation pays—even economically in terms of greatly reduced hospitalizations, let alone in terms of less suffering and new hope and a new lease on real life for the emphysemic. And there is every reason to believe that if rehabilitation can be provided earlier in the course of emphysema, we can make far greater inroads against the disease and its toll."

Overcoming Sensory Deprivation

One of the valuable contributions coming from space research has been the discovery that the same kind of mental deterioration which for long has been thought to be part of aging can be brought on not by age but by sensory deprivation. When denied normal, complex sensory stimulation—the sounds, sights, tastes, feel of the outer world and interaction with it and with people—even a healthy young person, space researchers determined, begins to show disorganized thinking ability.

In his book *Games People Play,* Dr. Eric Berne considered the need for stimuli and the probability that "emotional and sensory deprivation tends to bring about or encourage organic changes." He remarked that without sufficient stimulation degenerative changes in brain cells may occur, and that though "this may be a secondary effect due to poor nutrition . . . the poor nutrition itself may be a product of apathy . . . In this sense, stimulus hunger has the same relationship to survival of the human organism as food hunger."

Recognizing the need, some investigators have carried out promising studies even with clearly senile patients. One study was conducted by an educational consultant, a casework supervisor, and a recreational therapist in one of the senile wards of a home and hospital for the aged. The keynote of the program was sensory input to overcome the lack of stimuli for the patients. Because the medical staff was skeptical, the pilot program was confined to the twenty women in the one ward, all over eighty, needing constant physical care, confused, disoriented, withdrawn, depressed.

The team visited the ward daily, engaged the women in arts and crafts and handwork projects at bedside, and arranged for a twice-a-week live musical program with piano and guitar and with patients singing along, dancing, or clapping. Once a week, too, short movies were shown or bingo played, and a day was set aside for recorded music while giant balloons were tossed and bounced to the rhythm.

After six months, the patients showed marked improvement in many areas, including recognition, recall, overall behavior, and relationships with staff, relatives, and one another. Subsequently, the staff of other wards requested similar programming.

The same success has been reported from Australia, with "stimulation therapy" over a six-month period for women patients with senile dementia.

Even lesser sensory deprivation can be important in the elderly. "Sensory deprivation, often caused by decreased hearing or visual acuity, may add to the elderly person's preoccupation with his own mental production and decreases his ability for reality testing," report Drs. J. D. Hoogerbeets and John LaWall of the University of Arizona School of Medicine.

Hearing. Older people often suffer from hearing loss. But, as many have discovered, shouting at an elderly deaf person does no good, only causing low-frequency sounds to boom without increasing audibility of higher-frequency consonants, which is why so many older people protest, "Don't shout; I can hear," when, in fact, they do not understand what they hear.

Many people in their seventies and eighties do not necessarily have a flat loss in all frequencies. In fact, the two lowest frequencies are often useful but the higher ones may be useless. As a result, hearing may be fair for the lower vowel sounds but poor for upper frequencies, which include consonant sounds needed to differentiate words. For example, "fog" and "hog" may sound like "og."

As a result, many older people become "tuned out" of their social environment, with a resulting strong emotional impact that increases tension, agitation, or depression.

Often, the aged with hearing difficulties can be helped significantly by hearing aids; but those aids have to be very carefully, and expertly, chosen, with great patience often needed by both patient and specialist. Too often, otologists refer patients with problems not amenable to treatment to commercial dealers for a hearing aid rather than evaluating themselves all possible suitable hearing aids and selecting the best. Such otologists feel that there are no significant differences in individual hearing-aid performance.

But there can be great differences. In their experience with 6000 hard-of-hearing patients, Baylor University specialists found that often the first five or more aids were all uniformly poor in performance; but then, finally, one aid was found that produced excellent results. In many cases, they had to test ten or more aids to find one satisfactory for a particular patient.

In another study with 298 patients, Dr. O. Haug and other Houston investigators selected hearing aids, several for each patient, that theoretically, on the basis of the characteristics of the aids and the needs of the patients, should have provided peak performance.

But in actual use there were marked differences in effectiveness. In almost half (47 percent) of the patients, there were differences of 20 percent or more in speech discrimination between what proved to be for them the poorest and best performing aids. In 86 percent of the patients, there were differences of 10 percent or more.

Such considerable differences, the study suggests, justify the effort and expense involved in carefully evaluating various aids for an individual patient rather than letting it go at merely choosing an aid that theoretically should be suitable.

Nor is it always a matter of need for a hearing aid. In a special report on hearing problems in older people, Dr. Robert J. Ruben, professor and chairman of the Department of Otolaryngology of Albert Einstein College of Medicine, New York City, has pointed to many problems that are amenable to treatment.

Among the most easily treatable causes of hearing loss is wax that blocks the outer ear canal. Generally, this produces only a modest loss, but if there already is other loss, as Dr. Ruben puts it, "the combined impediment may stifle communication." Yet removal of wax can be carried out readily with a wax curette or by irrigation.

Other treatable causes include infection and reactions to drugs—even aspirin in some cases. Patients using large amounts of aspirin for arthritis who become sensitive to the drug and suffer hearing loss often regain the hearing when aspirin is stopped and another drug substituted. There are other causes which are amenable to treatment by surgery; and, as Dr. Ruben notes, surgery "can be successful in the elderly."

Vision. Three diseases—cataracts, macular disease, and glaucoma—or a combination of them account for the vast majority of eye problems in older people. Yet much can be done now to preserve and restore useful vision.

Cataracts are opaque spots that form on the lens of the eye and interfere with passage of light rays. Often the first indications are blurring and dimming of vision. Gradually the patient needs a brighter reading light or must hold objects closer to the eyes. Continued lens clouding may sometimes cause double vision.

Many elderly people are anxious both about cataracts and treatment for them, often because they do not understand the nature of the problem and its correction.

Advances in cataract removal procedures have made removal comparatively easy for the aged and infirm. No longer is there a period of immobilization that used to be required—erroneously.

Cataract removal can be carried out under local anesthesia.

Through an incision where the clear cornea and white of the eye meet, the lens is reached. It can then be loosened by an enzyme injection that dissolves the ligaments holding the lens without affecting other eye structures. The lens then can be lifted out readily and the incision closed. Many surgeons now allow patients out of the bed the day after.

Glasses are needed to replace the lens. Although they have thick lenses that make objects appear larger, most people adapt to them well. Instead of glasses, contact lenses may be used.

In macular disease, the macular area of the retina, which permits perception of fine detail such as print, degenerates, causing loss of central vision and ability to read and make out detail.

When the disease stems from inflammation, cortisonelike drugs may help, since they have anti-inflammatory effects. Even some noninflammatory cases respond to the drugs, possibly because they also remove excess fluid from the retina.

Macular disease is usually progressive. Yet, even when it has progressed to a marked degree, many older patients can be helped by prescriptions for special low-vision aids—magnifying devices available in hand-held form and also incorporated into eyeglass lenses.

Glaucoma, a major cause of blindness, affects about 10 percent of people by age sixty-five. Yet the disease can be arrested when detected and treated early in its course.

Inside the front of the eye, the aqueous humor, a circulating fluid is formed continuously and normally drains off so the same fluid pressure is maintained. In glaucoma, drainage of the fluid is impeded, pressure builds up, inhibiting blood supply and after a time damaging nerve cells.

The damage, starting at the edges, slowly moves toward the center. The victim loses side vision and develops "tunnel vision," viewing objects as though through a telescope. There may also be blurring of vision and rainbow-colored rings may be seen around lights.

There are many varieties of glaucoma, but all have in common increased pressure within the eyeball because fluid does not drain properly. Most often, glaucoma is sneaky, developing slowly and painlessly, and producing no symptoms until damage is done. Yet the warning elevation of pressure can be detected readily by a physician using a tonometer, a pressure-sensing instrument.

Often, eyedrops help, controlling production of aqueous humor or facilitating drainage so pressure is reduced toward normal. If eyedrops are inadequate, surgery may be used. In one procedure, a small segment of the iris—the colored part of the eye around the pupil—is cut off, leaving a small, almost invisible opening that allows increased drainage. The procedure can be done under local or general anesthesia and the patient is out of bed within a day or two.

An alternative operation is sclerectomy. A tiny hole is made in the outer coat of the eye, into the space under the sclera, which is the outer white eyeball sheath. Without leaving a visible scar, this provides a new fluid drainage channel.

Surgery for glaucoma is delicate but not life-threatening.

Never Too Old for Surgery

When a ninety-one-year-old man was admitted to a New York City hospital, the outlook seemed grim. He was very sick. Over six feet tall, he weighed only 110 pounds, complained of great weakness and breathing difficulty. Examination showed that he had abnormal heart sounds, lung congestion, gallstones, a severe groin hernia, and a large scrotal mass.

For ten days, his heart and lung conditions were treated medically and he was nourished to build up his strength. Then, in a single session at the operating table, surgeons carried out multiple procedures. They removed his gallbladder and immediately, through another incision, pulled his protruding, herniated bowel back into the abdominal cavity. They then repaired the hernia and took care of the scrotal mass. He went home seventeen days later, free of all complaints.

An exceptional case? It shouldn't be.

Elderly people, it has become clear, are not as delicate as many people—and many physicians as well—have thought. They can tolerate extensive surgery and benefit from it.

A sharply pointed editorial in the *Journal of the American Medical Association* not long ago noted a considerable body of evidence that surgery for older people has become increasingly safe and often able to produce improvement in the quality of life. It drew a parallel between an age for mandatory retirement from work and "mandatory retirement from therapy"—denial of major surgery.

The journal criticized "the underlying assumption that the quality of life attainable in the elderly is poor at best, so that heroic attempts at improving handicaps and disabilities are hardly worthwhile."

The new perception about older people encompasses many kinds of operations.

When he was seventy-six, Averell Harriman, elder statesman and a former governor of New York, underwent successful surgery for hernia. Yet it wasn't very long ago, as one of America's most distinguished surgeons, Dr. Alton Ochsner of New Orleans' Ochsner Clinic, recalls, when an operation for a hernia for anyone even older than fifty was considered unjustified. Currently, 98 percent successful repair rates are being reported in patients over seventy, even in those over ninety, including some with life-threatening strangulation obstruction.

Serious diverticular disease—involving severely inflamed, extremely painful, and often life-threatening colon outpouchings—has its greatest incidence in older people. When surgery is essential, is it too risky? At St. Vincent's Hospital and Medical Center, New York City, in 370 patients the overall operative death rate was 4.4 percent for those over seventy and 2.5 percent for those under seventy. But with a special procedure called a three-stage operation, there were no deaths in patients over seventy.

Gallbladder surgery? In one recent large study, aged patients were found to have a 98 percent chance for recovery. Among the patients in the study was a seventy-two-year-old woman who needed more than gallbladder removal. A dangerously ballooned section (aneurysm) of her aorta, the main artery from the heart, had to be replaced with a graft, and a threatening clot had to be removed from a leg artery. She came through it all nicely.

In a suburban hospital, an elderly woman presented a seemingly insuperable problem. She was in agonizing pain. A diseased abdominal artery was obstructing blood flow to her small intestine, which had become gangrenous. She had to have massive surgery—removal of all but eighteen inches of her small bowel. Yet eleven years later, she was alive and well.

One reported study after another has been revealing that when various cancers—colon, lung, prostate, and others—are surgically treatable, patients in their seventies and even older respond well.

The aortic valve regulates blood flow from the heart to the whole body. Narrowing of the valve (stenosis) makes blood pumping difficult for the heart and may lead to chest pain and easy fatigability. Although surgery to replace the valve has helped many middle-aged and younger patients, there has been reluctance to resort to operation for the elderly for fear that age increases the risk. But a recent National Institutes of Health study indicates that age in itself no longer can be regarded as a reason not to operate.

Seventy-three patients, aged sixty to seventy-seven, who underwent valve replacement were compared with 277 who had surgery at ages twelve to fifty-nine. The hospital death rate in the elderly was actually only half that of the younger patients, the later death rate was no higher, and the improvement in both groups was nearly identical.

Surgery for younger patients with coronary heart disease—suffering chest pain and at risk of heart attack because adequate blood for the heart muscle cannot get through choked-up coronary arteries—uses vein grafts to bypass blocked artery sections. Pain often is greatly relieved, and risk of heart attack may be reduced. Over-sixty-five patients undergoing such surgery do almost as well as younger patients. In one study of persons aged seventy and over, more than 90 percent came through the operation well.

Recently, a concerned family sought help for an elderly woman with severe parkinsonism, or shaking palsy, who also had begun to suffer mental deterioration. Fortunately, when told by one physician that there was nothing to be done and the patient would have to get alone as well as she could, the family insisted on consultation. Thorough neurological studies revealed a brain tumor. The tumor was removed successfully. Almost immediately the parkinsonism disappeared. Not long afterward, the mental dullness was gone. Rehabilitation was complete.

Certainly, hasty, ill-advised, or needless surgery is wrong for anyone, young or old. But it is also wrong to deny needed surgery simply because of age—or because of a sometimes misguided notion that it is better to allow an elderly patient to "die with dignity."

Among surgical procedures used routinely for younger people which could also benefit afflicted elderly are the stripping of varicose veins to restore adequate blood circulation and avoid unyielding leg ulcers; the removal of hemorrhoids; the repair of dropped wombs, bladders, and rectal tissue; the repair of hernias and removal of enlarged prostates; the reattachment of detached retinas and treatment of glaucoma and cataract; and the sometimes-possible reversal of progressive hearing loss.

Surgical advances have been catching up with advancing age. What's needed, along with appreciation of that fact, is appreciation of another: that there can and should be a richer quality of life for the elderly, and that surgery, when indicated, often can help make it possible.

13

The Matter of Vigor

Several years ago, in a report to the U.S. Senate, Senator Jennings Randolph told of a demonstration he had witnessed in some amazement in Charlestown, West Virginia, while conducting hearings for the Senate Committee on Aging.

He had observed a group of elderly people go through vigorous exercises. All had suffered from chronic conditions or had been recovering from acute physical disabilities which had almost completely immobilized them.

Yet, within six months after becoming participants in a Physical Fitness for Senior Citizens program of the Lawrence Frankel Foundation in Charlestown, they were no longer relegated to the sidelines.

A seventy-two-year-old woman who had broken both legs, had been informed by physicians she might never walk again, and had spent three years in a residence home was moving freely. An eighty-one-year-old man, incapacitated totally for two years after a spinal operation, now could walk unassisted. A sixty-nine-year-old woman, long ill with heart disease, spinal arthritis, and a nerve ailment, needing sleeping pills nightly, now could do sit-ups and strength exercises, balance on a beam, and needed no sleeping pills since starting the program.

Almost at the same time came striking case reports from the University of Southern California's Gerontology Center, where 150 older people are taking part in a long-range study on the

189

practicality and usefulness of exercise in the elderly.

One of the participants, a businessman, had suffered through much of his adult life with severe migraine attacks. Nothing had seemed to help. At the age of sixty-seven, six weeks after starting on a Center-prescribed program of exercises, his headaches vanished. Rarely in his life had he worked up a sweat. But the exercise program he follows now makes him feel so good he carries it on out of doors even when it's raining.

Another participant, the eighty-seven-year-old retired president of the Union Theological Seminary in the Philippines, engages in jogging three times a week and has found it "has made a much younger man out of me."

What these and other studies and experiences are establishing is the falsity of a whole series of assumptions about the elderly: that aging must inevitably bring rapid physical decline which is neither preventable nor remediable; that older people are incapable of vigorous activity, which can even be dangerous for them, harmful rather than helpful.

And on the positive side, what is being proved is that the elderly need to be active and can be; that they even have a special need for activity; and that suitable activity can lead to rehabilitation benefits even in some of the seemingly most hopeless cases of decline.

Reported Benefits

At the University of Wisconsin, Madison, Professor Everett Smith, a preventive medicine specialist, has been finding that while exercise is not a fountain of youth, it can help an elderly person be "better off" at each chronological age.

Although exercise cannot stop aging, it can increase a person's endurance, range of motion, and strength. Exercise, Smith reports, also can help maintain greater joint flexibility for up to 80 percent of arthritics. In addition, physical activity prevents bone demineralization and retards further progress of the degenerative diseases of aging. And a person sixty-five or over who is put on an exercise program, Smith emphasizes, can gain back at least 15 percent of his or her work capacity.

Late in 1977, the National Institute on Aging held a three-day seminar attended by experts from around the world. The subject: exercise in aging. And the experts, as one medical publication put it, "virtually certified exercise both as a prophylactic against and a remedy for rapid decline in the elderly."

As they reported, exercise among other things can help to compensate for declining heart and blood function with aging, keep lungs younger, reduce nervous system irritability, restore a youthful ratio of muscle to fat, and, in doing so, may restore more youthful rates of metabolism (the body's overall energy activities).

Clues

Only recently has the possible usefulness of exercise in older people—and its practicality for them—come in for intensive research.

It has been known, of course, that body activities and physiological processes tend to slow through the middle years and thereafter.

Commonly, the maximum rate at which the heart can operate slows—by about six beats per minute for each five years, beginning not long after age twenty-five. The amount of blood pumped by the heart with each beat or contraction also decreases. Meanwhile, blood pressure tends to increase, while breathing efficiency declines by as much as 25 percent. Bones, too, lose resiliency and become more fragile. The average man reaches his peak of muscular strength in the late teens, more or less maintains it up to about age forty-five, after which it declines about 15 percent by age sixty-five. A similar pattern applies for women, except that their strength peak comes with onset of puberty.

But how much of this decline is inevitable with aging? How much depends upon health practices, including physical activity, or lack of them?

One clue to the influence of lack of physical activity has been found in the fact that, at any age, young or old, enforced inactivity such as bed rest for a period of time produces many of the deteriorations seen in aging.

In one study, when researchers measured the effects of bed rest for a four-week period in healthy young men, they found a 17 percent decrease in heart volume, an 8 percent decrease in the heart's transverse diameter, and an increase in pulse rate of one beat per minute for each two days in bed.

In the first space flights, it was very quickly noted that astronauts experienced deteriorating effects which could be traced to lack of physical activity. In later flights, equipment for exercising was installed in spacecraft and exercise programs were prescribed.

Actually, more than a dozen years ago, Drs. Hans Kraus and Wilhelm Raab of New York University proposed a concept of "hypokinetic disease"—literally, diminished movement—which they considered to cover a broad spectrum of physical and mental derangements traceable to inactivity.

They noted that not only is coronary heart disease with its heart attack consequence more common in sedentary than in physically active people; so are diabetes, ulcers, and low back pain. They suggested that lack of physical exercise parallels emotional problems. They also saw the physically active as better adaptable to stress, and as having less tension, less fatigability, lower blood pressure, greater breathing capacity, more strength and flexibility. They also noted that active persons seem likely to age later.

But aren't the elderly basically incapable of vigorous physical performance?

To be sure, as one concerned physician, Dr. Gerald H. Pratt of the New York University School of Medicine, points out, "With increasing age, the individual becomes a follower of . . . the 'chair syndrome.' The patient sits rather than stands. Exercise and even walking is discontinued and replaced by rides even for short distances. To this chair habit can be added the lounge and, worst of all, the bed. Elderly persons elect or are relegated by well-intentioned relatives or friends to enforced inactivity. This regimen is encouraged in many homes or institutions to reduce the necessity of attendance or care. With these hours of inactivity the arterial and venous circulation slows and may even stop."

There are, of course, exceptions. The President's Council on Physical Fitness and Sports points to a woman who at age eighty-five and again at eighty-six won gold medals in half-mile and mile runs in "Senior Olympic" competition. Clarence DeMar, a celebrated distance runner, ran 1000 distance races, including 100 marathons, in his lifetime. At sixty-nine, he ran a fifteen-kilometer (almost ten-mile) race. For 94 of his 106 years, Larry Lewis, a San Francisco waiter, made it a practice to run six miles a day every day through Golden Gate Park.

Although generally older people cannot achieve performance levels equal to those attainable when they were younger, they are, the President's Council emphasizes, trainable; and not only can many body deteriorations be slowed, but some may even be reversible for longtime sedentary men and women.

At the University of Southern California, ninety-six volunteers aged sixty to eighty-seven participated in a study during which they exercised three times a week, cautiously at first, gradually increasing their activities. Even at the end of six weeks, they showed significant benefits, including a 6 percent drop in blood pressure and a 9 percent gain in "maximum oxygen uptake," a measurement which is considered to be a prime indicator of fitness.

In a recent investigation of the possible retarding effect of exercise on aging, San Diego State University researchers headed by Dr. Fred Kasch set out to determine if the 9 to 15 percent decline in physical work capacity usually experienced by men between the ages of forty-five and fifty-five could be altered. Over a ten-year period, a group of men who averaged 44.6 years of age at the start, averaged three days of workouts a week, twelve months of the year. Most ran, but one man swam and two combined running and swimming. The average running distance a week was fifteen miles.

Throughout the ten-year period, the men maintained relatively constant body weight, blood pressure, and breathing capacity and, in fact, improved their breathing efficiency. And, the investigators reported, sure enough, the usual 9 to 15 percent decline in work capacity was forestalled; indeed, the men showed a physical work capacity 25 percent greater than average.

At a recent National Institute on Aging seminar, Dr. Herbert de Vries reported on an exercise training program he has been conducting for the elderly at the Andrus Gerontology Center of the University of Southern California.

All subjects were sedentary to begin with. After a medical assessment, they started out the first day with limited activity—just jogging fifty paces and walking fifty paces, and repeating this five times. Gradually, the number of sets of jogging-walking was increased by one a day from five to a maximum of ten. Then, at that point, the number of jogging paces was held constant while the number of walking paces per set was reduced by ten a week, until in five weeks the participants were doing no more walking, only jogging. Thereafter, the jogging time was slowly increased.

Several precautions were carefully observed. Each training session began with a slow warm-up and ended with a cool-down period, in each of which the participants walked and stretched.

Among the elderly he has put into running shoes, Dr. de Vries reported, he has seen a 29 percent improvement in heart rate, vital capacity, and strength after forty-two weeks of the program.

There were also decreases in skin-fold thickness (a measure of body fat) and reductions in blood pressure. And a healthy tranquilizing effect was achieved—greater than among other older people actually receiving tranquilizing pills and without side effects.

There were other striking reports at the aging seminar:

- Dr. Richard Riley of Johns Hopkins University noted that lung changes with aging tend to be identical in kind although not in degree to those of the lung disease emphysema. Between age twenty-five and age seventy-five, there is a quart decrease in lung capacity, and the amount of stale air kept in the lungs instead of being exhaled increases. Yet, as a result of exercise training, lung function is improved.
- Dr. L. Howard Hartley of Harvard reported significant beneficial changes from exercise in endocrine gland hormones and nervous system hormones. He also has noted less irritability in people who exercise and lowered levels in the blood of lactate (a waste product), lowered heart rate, and greater blood flow to the kidneys and other body organs.
- Although a decline in aerobic capacity—the ability to carry out physical activities without having the body crave oxygen—occurs with age, the decline can be postponed by as much as twenty years by an exercise training program, reported Dr. Per-Olaf Astrand of Stockholm.
- Another beneficial effect of exercise, reported Dr. Jana Pariskova of Charles University in Prague, Czechoslovakia, is that it maintains a constant fat/lean body composition ratio, which otherwise, beginning around age thirty, shifts in favor of more fat and less lean.
- Considering the loss of muscle mass with aging among sedentary people, the long-held idea that the body's metabolic rate—the rate at which food can be converted into useful energy for body processes—must decline with age needs revision, reported Dr. Francisco Grande of Spain. The meta-

bolic rate decrease may in fact be an expression instead of the changes in body composition in the sedentary, since muscle has a higher metabolic rate than fat.

As one medical publication *(Medical Tribune)* aptly summed up these and other reports at the seminar: "Despite the differences in their specialties, most of the participants had the same basic message to deliver to physicians: Don't overestimate the inevitability of deterioration from aging and don't underestimate the ability of the elderly body to respond to reasonable demands."

Heart Protector

New insights into the role of inactivity in increasing risk of heart trouble and of exercise in reducing that risk have been coming recently.

One striking report was made to the National Institute on Aging seminar by Dr. Ralph Paffenberger of Stanford University Medical School based on his findings in a study of California longshoremen and their on-job activity and in another study of Harvard alumni and their leisure activities.

For both groups, Dr. Paffenberger found, the number of fatal heart attacks decreased as energy output increased.

Of the 3686 longshoremen studied, those in low-energy jobs, expending as few as 4750 calories a week, had a 50 percent higher risk than those burning more than 10,000 calories a week—and the sudden death rate was also three times higher in the low-energy group.

Among the 16,936 Harvard men ranging in age up to seventy-four who were carefully followed over a ten-year period by periodic questionnaires to elicit information on their health and on their exercising, sports participation, and other leisure-time activities, a similar relationship between exercise and reduced heart trouble risk was noted.

These results, Dr. Paffenberger reported, mean that inactivity has equal billing with smoking as a potent heart risk factor, outranking body weight, blood sugar, and blood cholesterol.

Actually, the role of exercise in regulating blood cholesterol has recently come in for a searching new look because of new findings about how cholesterol is handled in the body.

The fatty substance, of course, has long been associated, when present in high levels in the blood, with atherosclerosis, the artery-clogging disease responsible for the most important form of heart disease leading to invalidism and heart attacks.

Cholesterol, in fact, occurs in every body cell. The body itself produces it because it plays vital roles. For example, it is the material from which the sex hormones and the hormones of the adrenal glands, such as cortisone, are derived. It is also used to make the bile acids required for digestion.

Cholesterol is also taken in through diet, with foods such as egg yolk, butter, and lobster relatively high in it.

But now a fundamental new insight.

Fatty substances such as cholesterol do not mix with water, and so the blood cannot carry them. To transport cholesterol and other fats to various organs and tissues where they are needed, the body attaches them to proteins that have the ability to dissolve in the blood. Fats are known chemically as lipids, and the fat-protein combinations found in the blood are called lipoproteins.

What has been known for some time is that there is more than one kind of lipoprotein and that cholesterol is carried in two major types: high-density (HDL) and low-density (LDL) lipoproteins.

But the distinction got relatively little attention until 1977, when investigators in the government's famed Framingham study announced what has been called a "bombshell" discovery. The finding: that more important than total cholesterol in the blood is the ratio between HDL and LDL.

Studying new cases of coronary heart disease developing among the more than 5000 participants in the study in the Massachusetts community, all healthy to start, the investigators found low HDL levels in the great majority. And, in a corollary finding, it turned out that the higher the HDL levels, the less likelihood of heart trouble.

How does HDL protect?

It now appears that LDL is involved in carrying cholesterol to and depositing it in tissues, including artery walls, where its build-up impairs circulation and may lead to heart disease and heart attack. On the other hand, HDL does the opposite. It removes cholesterol from areas where it is in excess and carries it to the liver for disposal. So it appears that the protective effect of HDL lies in its ability to thwart the atherosclerotic process by removing cholesterol from artery walls.

Since HDL is protective, what can be done to increase its level in the blood? Some drugs—clofibrate and niacin, for example—have been found to increase the level. So, too, a diet emphasizing vegetables, cereals, fish, relatively little meat, and no foods such as hot dogs and potato chips, which are loaded with saturated fats.

But exercise also is effective, much more so than previously believed. Exercise has been known in the past to help bring down total cholesterol levels, but not to any dramatic degree.

Recently, however, Dr. Peter D. Wood and other Stanford University investigators checked a group of very active men who routinely ran at least fifteen miles a week. They were compared with other men of similar ages leading sedentary lives.

The runners had a cholesterol level overall of 200 versus a somewhat higher level for the other men. But, significantly, the runners had a much higher mean level of HDL.

"Thus," observes Dr. Alexander Leaf of Harvard Medical School, "physical activity in this study, as in others, was associated with only a small decrease in total cholesterol but with a

marked alteration in the distribution [of HDL]. So run and preserve your [healthy] profile of lipoproteins."

Heart Restorer

More than four million Americans now have cardiac disability,
according to some estimates. After recovery from a heart attack,
many people live half-lives, fearful of engaging in almost any
activity or exertion. Some have the capacity but are overpower-
ingly anxious; others have impaired capacity, and some even
have wasted-away muscles and decreased lung and breathing
functions.

Recently, many physicians have been demonstrating that much
can be done to restore these people to normal or near-normal
lives. And in a growing number of hospitals now, heart attack
victims, even while still in coronary care units, are encouraged
to become ambulatory. During the rest of hospitalization, physical activity is encouraged and increased systematically.

During convalescence at home, they are urged to return gradually to ordinary daily activities. Then, in a final phase of rehabilitation, they get exercise conditioning in programs often super-
vised in hospital outpatient departments, rehabilitation centers,
or community recreation facilities. The programs aim at helping
them reach optimum heart fitness levels so they become capable
of engaging in desired work and leisure activities.

In a report not long ago, Dr. Arthur S. Leon of the University
of Minnesota noted that significant increases in heart fitness
can be obtained with as few as three twenty- to thirty-minute
exercise sessions a week, with considerable improvement becoming evident within four weeks.

Moreover, Dr. Leon noted, there are important psychological
benefits from exercise programs, including "reduced mental depression and anxiety, improvement in self-confidence, and a return to feelings of well-being and good health."

And Psychological Benefits

Many investigations have been carried out among school- and college-age people to determine the psychological benefits of physical activity. More recently, some have been done in older people.

At Michigan State University, Dr. Henry Montoye has found that regular exercise increases the interest of older people in other people and the world about them, their energy for doing mental work, and in general their vigor for carrying out everyday activities.

In a study by Purdue University investigators, a check was made of personality differences among high fitness and low fitness groups of both young and older men. Using standard personality questionnaries, inventories and scales, the investigators found that the high fitness groups, both young and old, were more intellectually inclined, emotionally stable, composed, secure, easygoing, and adventurous than the low fit.

That exercise, in fact, can be useful therapy for emotional difficulties has been reported recently by many psychiatrists.

When Dr. Thaddeus Kostrubala of Mercy Medical Center, San Diego, a few years ago himself took up running, he also started a group of his psychiatric patients running three times a week. The changes in the patients, he has reported, have been remarkable. Those with depression had fewer symptoms; smoking and drinking were reduced or eliminated; personal relationships improved; even a schizophrenic patient could be taken off medication.

Dr. Kostrubala suggests that physical activity may possibly cause some body chemistry reaction that helps to restore emotional stability, or it may simply be a means by which patients can begin to take control of their lives again.

In one test of twenty-eight depressed patients, a University of Wisconsin Medical School team found that for most of them thirty to forty-five minutes of jogging three times a week was at least as effective as talk therapy.

Dr. Robert S. Brown of the University of Virginia at Charlottes-ville recalls thinking one day that nobody he had seen "jogging down at the track ever appeared depressed" and thereafter find-ing that exercise often works better than drugs in controlling depression. More than two-thirds of the patients he sees are depressives, and he has been finding that all but 15 to 20 percent of them show "quick benefit" after as little as a week of running. Dr. Brown's theory is that running fights depression by inducing desirable chemical changes in the brain, and he is currently work-ing with researchers at the National Institute of Mental Health to test the theory.

Even some years ago, Dr. Hans Selye of the University of Montreal, who developed the whole modern concept of stress and stress diseases, conducted a classic experiment with rats.

He subjected ten sedentary laboratory rats to a stressful course of deafening noise, blinding lights, and electric shocks to the point where in one month all ten were dead. Then he gave ten of their former cage-mates a course of exercise on a treadmill until they were in prime physical condition, after which he sub-jected them to the exact same series of stresses.

After a month of this torture, the second batch of rats were still alive, well, and thriving. The stresses deadly to the first rats were largely, as in man, psychological stresses. While the sedentary rats seemed to give up and die, the well-exercised rats apparently could withstand the stresses.

A Special Need of Older People

There may even be a special—and profound—need for and psychological value in exercise for older people, report two Is-raeli investigators, Drs. Hans and Sulomic Kreitler.

All of us, the Kreitlers note, start out enjoying movement—especially as children, when we relish movement just for the sake of moving. And that enjoyment of movement—in play, sports, dancing, and other activities—is common throughout adolescence and young adulthood.

But for sedentary older people, any pleasure derived from movement is steadily reduced, and eventually there develops a reluctance to move at all. Such inactivity not only promotes muscular degeneration, it also leads to psychological changes.

One of those changes is distortion of body image. Physically inactive older people, the Kreitlers report, often perceive their bodies to be heavier and broader than they really are, and because of this distorted perception they come to consider bodily movements increasingly difficult and strenuous.

A vicious cycle develops. Finding movements to be more and more effortful, older people often make less and less effort to move, and the restriction of activity adds still further to the body image distortion, which then results in greater clumsiness and fear of physical activity.

Other psychological effects then ensue. Without physical outlet for discharging energy, older people experience increased internal tension. The build-up of tension can produce varied symptoms—among them, fretfulness, restlessness, and sleeping difficulty. Subsequently, the elderly may turn inward on themselves, experiencing depression, which in turn may lead to physical disturbances as well.

Regular exercise for older people, according to the Kreitlers, can provide emotional satisfaction; it can break the cycle in which body image distortion caused by inactivity leads to more inactivity and further distortion; it can use up, in a healthy way, energies that need to be used up.

A Prescription for Exercise

Any sudden all-out effort—a vigorous burst of activity of any kind—can be dangerous for a long-sedentary person.

What is needed is a slow, cautious start after a careful physical checkup and medical advice.

Even mild activity can be valuable. In one study, for example, Dr. A. A. Kattus and associates at the University of California at Los Angeles worked with fifty people suffering from anginal chest pain associated with coronary heart disease. Patients were asked to walk increasing distances each day, but starting very modestly, with such distances as only one hundred feet three times a day. To do even that, some had to have nitroglycerin medication. Yet many of the people in the study reached the point of walking two miles a day, and in 75 percent of them the angina improved markedly.

Once mild activity produces benefits, the benefits may be increased by more vigorous activity, gradually arrived at.

One good model for an exercise program for older, long-sedentary people is that used by Dr. Herbert de Vries which was described earlier in this chapter.

It should be noted, too, that interested physicians today are in a position to provide valuable specific individual advice about exercise for older people.

Authorities, including the Committee on Exercise of the American Heart Association, have been developing guidelines for physicians to use in prescribing exercises as rationally as they can prescribe medication when required. Until recently, physicians, who usually had little training in exercise physiology, had little useful concrete advice to offer.

Heart rate can be an important guide. There are now standards for what the heart rate should be in various age groups. Physicians can employ those standards to help assure that exercise is beneficial without causing excessive strain.

Older people can be taught to take their own heart rate by taking their pulse at an artery in the wrist or at the side of the neck. By taking the pulse for fifteen seconds immediately after finishing exercise, a reasonably valid estimate of heart rate attained during the exercise can be made. And a record of this, made by the patient at each exercise session, can be used by the physician for his follow-up prescriptions of exercise intensity and duration.

14

The Right Help
When It's Needed

A professional publication for physicians, *Modern Medicine,* carries as a feature in each issue an angry letter urging that "Somebody DO Something." Not long ago, one such letter, by Dr. Fred B. Charatan of Syosset, New York, was "about the mistreatment of elderly patients."

"I'm angry about the aged," wrote Dr. Charatan. "Specifically, I'm angry about the way many of my colleagues treat their elderly patients. Can't you recall colleagues' comments, from medical school on, as if they were convinced they'd never grow old? Fogey, crock, geezer, and biddy are a few of the derogatory terms I've heard them use. I've also witnessed some of the following 'treatments':

"1. Impatience or not-so-benign neglect . . .

"2. Parroting 'It's just your age' with nary an attempt to find the underlying cause of symptoms . . .

"3. Feeding the elderly patient a new drug for each new symptom. In time, the patient may be taking over a dozen drugs, with correspondingly increased risks of side effects and incompatible drug interactions."

Some years ago, an American Medical Association committee on aging reported that after fifteen years of study it had been unable to find a single disease entity or mental condition that

204

is necessarily related to the passage of time.

Too long and often had the terms "aging" and "degeneration" been used interchangeably by medical men and in the medical literature. The terms, the committee declared, needed to be clearly distinguished. If degeneration occurred with age, it wasn't because of age per se.

Age should be no bar to good medical or surgical treatment, the committee declared, and gave a name to the kind of medical practice that barred such treatment: "condescension medicine."

Such medicine has been manifested in many ways. It has been at work when an elderly patient or his or her family has been concerned about growing apathy and confusion and failing memory, and when, seemingly sympathetic, the physician without making any real investigation has nodded and said to a family member, "I'm afraid we'll have to become reconciled to this. Nothing to be done, really . . . senility . . . brain changes."

It has been at work when a physician has tut-tutted an elderly patient's physical complaints with a "Now, there, there. We must all expect such problems as we grow old," or when a patient has had physical problems but has suffered unduly from them, possibly because of a remediable emotional problem about which the physician has done nothing because consciously or unconsciously he has considered the patient as just "an old crock."

Preconceptions have fostered condescension medicine. Dr. Theodore Linz of Yale tells a classic story about a seventy-six-year-old man who was hospitalized because of heart failure and complete disorientation. After the heart failure was controlled and that had improved circulation to the brain, he became oriented and rational.

But, because the seventy-six-year-old kept saying that as soon as he could go home, his mother would drive over to pick him up, his doctors thought it best to keep him hospitalized until they could get further improvement in his mental state.

"Then," observes Dr. Linz, "one day, somewhat to their chagrin, his mother of 95 drove over from a town some hundred miles away, accompanied by her 97-year-old sister, and took their little boy home."

I remember Dr. Edward Henderson, a distinguished physician very much interested in geriatrics, telling me about a sixty-eight-year-old friend hospitalized after a heart attack. The patient also was a personal friend of the doctor in the hospital taking care of him. The next morning, Henderson asked how the patient was and his physician said, "Pretty bad. He has anuria [suppression of urine excretion] and I'm afraid he is going out."

Had there been any urological examination, any attempt to drain urine with a tube? No, there had not been, Henderson discovered, possibly because of a defeatist attitude: The man was elderly and, with a heart attack, appeared doomed, and nothing else mattered.

Yet, Henderson pointed out, he knew that the man had an enlarged prostate and prostate inflammation and that a urological examination was warranted. Very quickly, the examination was carried out, 1000 cubic centimeters of urine was removed by tube, and with proper treatment the patient recovered and went home.

Condescension medicine for older people has had many sources. The medical needs of the elderly have been generally neglected in medical training in the past. When a few years ago a Senate Special Committee on Aging investigated, it could find no mention at all of the subject in the catalogues of more than half of the nation's medical schools. Ironically, medical students received plenty of training in exotic diseases which most of them would never see in practice but little training in treating the elderly with whom they would be dealing every day.

Moreover, in the past there has been heavy emphasis in medicine on the diagnosis and treatment of acute illness, and great satisfaction for physicians in the fact that such illnesses often respond dramatically to treatment. But problems in the elderly are often chronic in nature, do not respond as dramatically, and little attempt was made to instill the concept that there was satisfaction to be gained from less spectacular improvement.

Hopeful Developments

Fortunately, the poor quality of medical care for the elderly and the need for drastic changes to improve the quality are being recognized.

And there *is* action.

It includes efforts by medical students to change the medical education system. Late in 1977, Doug Outcalt, medical student at the University of Arizona and president of the American Medical Student Association, an organization of more than 20,000 medical students, published an editorial in the association's journal, *The New Physician.*

Among Outcalt's pointed comments:

"The exposure most medical students do receive to the elderly is usually negative. We are led to believe that working with the elderly is depressing, time-consuming, and unrewarding. We . . . often see those in their later years go without diagnostic and therapeutic measures because their illness is falsely attributed to 'old age.'

"All of these learned attitudes later manifest themselves in the poor quality of health care received by the elderly. Pelvic and rectal exams are often deferred in the elderly, even though they are the group most likely to benefit from such procedures. Most physicians are unable to differentiate between a treatable psychotic depression and organic brain syndrome. Many treatable diseases, such as TB, appendicitis, hyperthyroidism and myocardial infarction, often present differently in the elderly and frequently are missed in diagnosis. Many drugs have longer half-lives in older patients . . . yet dosages often are not reduced and corresponding side effects are attributed to the age of the patient and ignored. Proper orientation to the elderly patient could eliminate all of these common errors.

"Fortunately, the voices calling for a change in the approach medical education has taken toward the elderly are growing louder. A few scattered geriatricians are succeeding in opening the eyes of medical educators to the needs of the elderly. Elderly consumer groups are beginning to demand more and better services, and, most importantly, students are beginning to realize a deficiency in their educations and are asking to be taught all that is needed to become a high quality, complete physician.

"The time is right for us to provide the impetus for starting courses in geriatrics at all medical schools. These courses should emphasize all that is positive and rewarding about treating and working with older patients and should teach us to deal competently and humanely with them."

Within a few months, the AMSA had established a Task Force on Aging to press for such courses.

There are many other indications of a changing climate:

- An American Medical Association publication, *Impact,* recently surveyed practicing physicians and found that 75 percent answered yes to the question "Do MD's need special training in geriatrics?"
- The Veterans Administration in July 1978 began a geriatrics training program for physicians at six of its hospitals which are affiliated with medical schools.
- The first endowed chair in geriatrics in the country has been established at Cornell University Medical College.
- A bill to provide financial grants for geriatric education in medical schools recently was introduced into the U.S. Senate (S. 2287).
- The Ohio State Legislature recently enacted a bill calling for each of the seven medical schools in the state to set up "an office within a department, or a department" of geriatric medicine immediately, with funds allotted to help.

- The American Geriatrics Society, which began with only 352 members about twenty-five years ago, now numbers more than 7000 physicians.
- A considerable number of reports devoted to the diagnosis and treatment of problems of older people—and to research directed at new insights—now appear in the medical literature.
- Hospital residency training programs have been established at the Oak Forest (Illinois) Hospital and at the Jewish Institute for Geriatric Care, which is part of the Long Island Jewish–Hillside Medical Center in New Hyde Park, New York. And other hospitals are beginning to show interest in establishing such residency programs.

The goal of the program at the Jewish Institute for Geriatric Care, which is directed by Dr. Leslie S. Libow, is to train physicians to act as coordinators of a team approach in caring for the elderly. Included in the team are representatives of every specialty that may be needed to treat an aged patient, from the ophthalmologist who removes cataracts to the orthopedist who will set a broken hip.

The Institute provides not only treatment in the hospital when that is needed but also outpatient-clinic care and the services of a visiting nurse and resident physicians who make house calls. Staff members provide or arrange for social services and other home care services.

In its first six years, the Institute has had more applicants among physicians to become residents than it could accept. More than 150 medical students from sixteen medical schools have studied there in four- to eight-week clinical clerkships.

Many of those who were trained as residents now have become directors of geriatric programs at medical schools and hospitals around the country. One of them, interestingly, Dr. Albert A. Fisk, was in medical practice for twenty years and was a board-certified internist and chief of staff at an Ohio hospital before deciding to take a geriatric residency. He has since become direc-tor of the Wisconsin Regional Geriatric Center, a program in Milwaukee set up jointly by Mount Sinai Medical Center and Family Hospital.

One example of the kind of salutary experience residents in training and young medical students serving clinical clerkships get at the Institute: An old man who became a patient there was, when he was brought in, a pitiful sight. He could only slump in a chair. His eyelids drooped, his hands trembled, he wore no fewer than three sweaters to keep warm, and mumbled unintelligibly in response to questions.

Doctors at a major New York hospital had diagnosed his case as "possible stroke complicated by senility," and had written him off as hopeless.

But physicians at the Institute refused to write him off. The three sweaters provided a clue for the experts. A blood test quickly confirmed their suspicion: At eighty-one, the old man was suffering from an acute thyroid deficiency, in which low body heat is a major symptom. With daily thyroid hormone, his "senility" cleared dramatically and he could go home.

Where to Turn

Finally, the misguided long-held notion that "you just can't do much for older people" is being replaced by a true concep-tion: that much, indeed, can be done.

Almost certainly, you can count on a burgeoning of medical and allied personnel interested and specially trained in caring for older people. You can count, too, on a burgeoning of facili-ties—hospital departments, day care centers, and others—de-voted to vigorous efforts to properly diagnose and treat the problems of the elderly.

If you need help now—for yourself or for an elderly member of the family—you may be lucky enough to live in or near a community with a special facility to which you can turn for that help.

If not, perhaps there is available a physician who has had special training in a geriatric residency—or another physician, who may be an internist or family doctor, who takes an interest in problems of the elderly and may even have taken courses in aspects of geriatric care as part of his continuing medical education (as more and more physicians are doing). A local hospital, the county medical society, or perhaps your family physician may be able to direct you to such a physician.

No one physician can handle all the health problems of the elderly any more than he can all those of younger people. But he should, first of all, be seriously interested in the problems of older people, in finding solutions for them if possible, with a conviction that making the effort to find the solutions is worthwhile. And he should be willing and even eager to call in consultants for those problems he may suspect are at the root of trouble and in which he is not expert.

He should be a physician with whom the patient can communicate well, who takes care to get a full history, who explains what the problem is and makes every effort to be certain that the patient understands. Aware of the possibility that an older person may be suffering from more than one disorder at a time, he should be concerned about diagnosing and treating all that may be present. He should be concerned about any drugs he prescribes or the patient may already be using—monitoring carefully for suitable dosages and for patient compliance.

Finally, if you have any reason to suspect that possibly a problem described in this book may be applicable, you can ask your family physician to consider that possibility and, if necessary, recommend a neurologist, ophthalmologist, orthopedist, or other suitable specialist who may help.

15

The Frontiers

There has been research into aging and senility in the past, but not at all proportional to their importance. Recently, however, there has begun to be an intensification of investigational efforts—in government, university and medical center facilities, and in pharmaceutical laboratories.

The very young National Institute on Aging,* established in 1975, is playing an important role through studies in its own laboratories and research centers and research it sponsors elsewhere.

Although it would take many volumes to go fully into all of the investigational efforts currently under way, we can look here at some of the more promising highlights.

---

* The NIA was authorized by the Research on Aging Act signed into law on May 31, 1974. According to the Act:

The Congress finds and declares that—(1) the study of the aging process, the one biological condition common to all, has not received research support commensurate with its effects on the lives of every individual;

(2) in addition to the physical infirmities resulting from advanced age, the economic, social, and psychological factors associated with aging operate to exclude millions of Americans from the full life and the place in our society to which their years of service and experience entitle them;

(3) recent research efforts point the way toward alleviation of the problems of old age by extending the healthy middle years of life;

(4) there is no American institution that has undertaken comprehensive systematic and intensive studies of the biomedical and behavioral aspects of aging and the related training of necessary personnel;

(5) the establishment of a National Institute on Aging within the National Institutes of Health will meet the need for such an institution.

A Nootropic Era?

About twenty-five years ago came the first psychotropic agents—tranquilizers and other compounds for schizophrenia and other severe psychic illnesses that helped to make possible treatment instead of mere institutional warehousing.

Now we appear to be witnessing the beginnings of what could be another important development—of nootropic (mind-activating) agents. Such agents are aimed at the cognitive problems of older people—failing memory, slowing of thought processes, difficulty in concentrating and thinking clearly, even confusion.

Currently, in a growing number of special programs at major medical centers, elderly volunteers with such problems are joining investigators in many projects to evaluate innovative potential treatment measures coming out of pharmaceutical and other laboratories.

Among the first to operate have been programs at New York University Medical Center in New York City, Boston State Hospital, UCLA Medical Center in Los Angeles, and Long Island Jewish–Hillside Medical Center, New Hyde Park, New York. Still others are expected to open.

In some programs, volunteers pay a modest fee; in some, no fee at all; in all, they receive thorough examinations for any possible correctable physical problems—such as high blood pressure, vitamin deficiencies, metabolic disturbances, hydrocephalus, chronic infections—that could be contributing to cognitive troubles. And in the absence of any of these problems, they participate in the trials of innovative measures.

Depression, as we've seen earlier, is a common cause of cognitive troubles and what can seem to be senility. Many depressed elderly respond well to available antidepressant drugs. But for some, treatment with the available agents may be difficult or impossible because of possible effects on the heart in the presence of a heart problem.

Now pharmaceutical laboratories are beginning to develop new experimental antidepressants that they hope will have no undesirable effects for the elderly and can be useful for more of them.

One such agent currently under study is called Trazadone. It is still early in the trials, but indications are that it may be at least as effective as older antidepressants, without their side effects. Among other similar new agents under study at the various centers are Vivalan and Mianserin.

Among other types of drugs that have been used to try to help older people, as we have noted earlier, are vasodilators such as Hydergine and Cyclospasmol. Possibly, because they dilate or expand blood vessels, they could increase nourishing blood flow to brain tissues. And there have been reports of benefits to some patients—some relief of confusion, improvement in mental alertness and memory, increase in sociability.

Yet benefits, when they occurred with some vasodilators, did not always correlate well with increased blood flow. It appears that not all vasodilators are alike and that dilation may be only one effect, and not necessarily the prime effect, of some. There are indications that some may improve the brain's use of oxygen and nutrients and that some may help in specific instances to restore a proper chemical balance needed for normal nerve transmission.

Newer drugs of the vasodilator class are being developed and studied with the hope they will have definable effects that can be useful for more patients. One of those currently being evaluated at several centers is called Praxilene.

Another whole new area of research has been opened with the discovery that some hormones have effects on learning and behavior.

At the University of Utrecht in the Netherlands, Dr. David de Wied has been working with the hormone ACTH. Produced by the pituitary gland at the base of the brain, ACTH has long been known to serve as a stimulator for the adrenal glands atop the kidneys to release their hormones in times of stress.

Dr. de Wied split up the ACTH molecule and obtained a fraction called ACTH 4–10. He then experimented with it in animals. After training rats to go through a maze, he subjected them to electroshock to disrupt their memory. Some of the rats then received injections of ACTH 4–10 while others, for comparison, received injections of inert material. Those given the inert material had to learn to get through the maze all over again; those receiving 4–10 remembered immediately.

Early studies with ACTH 4–10 at some of the centers indicate that it may have a promising effect in facilitating memory retrieval in older people who often complain, "I know that; I just can't recall it." Some volunteers receiving 4–10 have also reported another effect: they feel much better generally after an injection.

Dr. de Wied has also produced a compound, 2766, related to ACTH 4–10, which can be given by mouth instead of by injection; and 2766 is now under study at some of the centers.

Recently, too, de Wied has found that vasopressin, another pituitary hormone, long known to function in the control of blood pressure and body water balance, plays a part in memory. Some European studies with vasopressin in human patients indicate possible benefits, and studies are expected to begin here.

"Brain Food"

An increasing number of degenerative brain diseases are being found to be associated with abnormal levels of certain neurotransmitters—substances secreted by brain cells to carry impulses to other brain cells.

And there is now considerable hope—and even some precedent—that restoring those levels to normal may improve faulty memory and cognition in affected older people.

Shaking palsy (Parkinson's disease), for example, is a degenerative brain disorder which is associated with low levels of a neurotransmitter called dopamine. A drug used successfully to relieve symptoms of that disorder is L-dopa. L-dopa is a precursor for dopamine, a material from which the neurotransmitter is produced.

Many cells in the brain use another neurotransmitter called acetylcholine. And there is a growing body of evidence that such cells are involved in memory and other important brain functions. There is also recent evidence suggesting that a deficiency of acetylcholine may underlie memory impairment and possibly some other changes that may occur with aging. Such evidence raises the possibility that treatment with materials that might increase the availability of brain acetylcholine might also alter the undesirable changes.

Choline, which goes into the making of acetylcholine, is not produced by brain cells. Instead, it must be obtained from the blood, which receives a small amount of it from the liver and the rest from lecithin, a choline-containing constituent of eggs, soybeans, liver, and other foods.

At Massachusetts Institute of Technology, a research group headed by Dr. Richard J. Wurtman discovered that on an hour-to-hour basis the amount of the neurotransmitter acetylcholine in the brain seems to depend on how much choline-rich food an individual has eaten recently.

Dr. Edith Cohen, then an MIT graduate student, was able to show in experimental animals that increases in levels of choline in the blood produced by injecting choline or by providing it in the diet caused major increases in brain choline and acetylcholine levels.

Within four months after the MIT workers reported that choline administration increases brain acetylcholine levels in animals, a medical use was suggested. Drs. Kenneth L. Davis, Philip A. Berger, and Leo E. Hollister, a psychiatric team at Stanford University, reported marked improvement after choline administration in a patient suffering from tardive dyskinesia.

Tardive dyskinesia is a disease which causes uncontrollable

movements of the tongue, mouth, face, and upper trunk. It is a common side effect that develops in many mental patients under regular treatment with powerful antipsychotic tranquilizing agents. In some patients it persists long after treatment with the drugs. Similar disorders also have been seen in some aged patients with no history of taking antipsychotic drugs.

Investigators had suspected for several years that tardive dyskinesia resulted from the release of inadequate amounts of acetylcholine in the brain. But no drug was available to restore the neurotransmitter.

The Stanford report, indicating the possible value of choline, was followed by studies carried out by Dr. Wurtman and his colleagues which confirmed the value. When they treated a group of patients suffering from chronic tardive dyskinesia for two weeks with choline and, for comparison, two weeks with a placebo (a look-alike but inert preparation), many patients showed major improvement after choline but none responded at all to the placebo.

Now studies are under way at MIT and elsewhere on the possible uses of choline—or lecithin—to treat an array of other diseases believed to involve acetylcholine deficiency, including memory loss and depression.

Meanwhile, other promising studies are under way using other approaches to the acetylcholine neurotransmission system.

Cholinesterase is an enzyme present in the brain which under some circumstances usefully breaks down and inactivates acetylcholine. It is possible that an excess of the enzyme might interfere with normal neurotransmitter activity. And, in fact, small doses of chemicals that can inhibit cholinesterase have been reported to facilitate maze learning in laboratory animals.

Physostigmine is one such enzyme inhibitor. Recently the drug was found to enhance both storage and retrieval of information in a woman with profoundly impaired cognitive function.

And, subsequently, investigators at the Veterans Administration Hospital, Palo Alto, California, studied physostigmine in normal healthy volunteers, administering one milligram of the drug by slow intravenous infusion one day and, for comparison, administering one milligram of an inert solution another day. The drug did, indeed, significantly enhance long-term memory storage and retrieval.

Almost at the same time, investigators at the National Institute of Mental Health and St. Elizabeths Hospital, Washington D.C., were also finding, in normal human subjects, that not only choline but another compound, arecoline, enhanced learning.

It should be emphasized that much study remains to be done before there can be any practical wide-scale application of choline, arecoline, physostigmine, or other agents under investigation. They may or may not turn out to be really useful for overcoming or preventing cognitive disorders and senility.

But, considering that only a few years ago it seemed highly improbable that any external influences could be applied to processes deep within the brain, the results of current research hold out great promise for eventually finding practical therapeutic and preventive measures.

Looking into the Basics

Why do people, in fact, age? Why do older people experience more illness? What are the underlying processes? Can any of those processes be manipulated for the better?

Aging, if it is the most universal of all biological phenomena, has probably been the least understood.

A growing volume of research now is trying to penetrate the mysteries. It is multifaceted—concerned with thoroughly evaluating through careful observation how people age and concerned, too, with studies at levels down through hormones and the cell receptors for hormones, the body immunity system, and the genes.

Actually, an important Longitudinal Study of Aging, which has been going on since 1958 at what is now the National Institute on Aging's Gerontology Research Center, adjoining the Baltimore City Hospitals, predates the NIA.

The study periodically examines 650 men between the ages of twenty and ninety-five to monitor heart, kidney, and lung function, body composition, exercise, physiology, carbohydrate and fat metabolism, drug handling, nutrition and endocrine factors, and behavioral and social variables. There are now plans to include women in the longitudinal study.

Because of the long-term nature of the study, only recently are some—by no means all—results coming from it. Some of the study observations are reflected in some of the information noted earlier, particularly in Chapter 2.

Among the findings of the study, for example: While older people may be as active as younger ones, they expend less energy in the process; with aging, there is a tendency to replace muscle with fat; lung function declines, but after age seventy there is leveling off of this decline; up to age fifty-five, on the average, cholesterol in the blood tends to increase, but thereafter there is a tendency for the level to decline, and older people may be at less risk of heart attack from this factor than younger people.

Much more is yet to come from the longitudinal study—all of it of great potential value in enabling researchers to more knowledgeably focus on problems to be solved, some of it of possible immediate practical value for physicians in treatment.

Another Gerontology Research Center area of investigation that holds promise concerns receptors. Hormones, of course, have long been known to be messenger chemicals. Circulating in the blood, they signal cells to carry out different activities at the right time—activities such as responding to stress and even to metabolizing foods.

Only recently, however, have investigators been able to determine how hormones pass on their messages to cells. They do so through receptors: tiny bodies of protein on the walls of cells.

And they have established that the receptors can be altered

under certain conditions—that, for example, they may be decreased by obesity and blocked by diabetes.

It occurred to Dr. George Roth and a team of researchers that hormone receptors might also be affected by aging. And they have, indeed, found changes in receptors—in laboratory animal studies (mice, rats, dogs) and in human studies. Receptor concentrations have been found to decrease with increasing age. Among the cells examined have been those of brain, liver, skeletal muscle, prostate, and lymphocytes (a type of white blood cell).

"We feel that this loss of receptors is an important mechanism in the aging process," says Dr. Roth.

And he and his colleagues are now trying to determine why the receptors decrease in number. There are several possibilities. One is that since the receptors normally are manufactured and broken down in the life cycle of a cell, they may possibly be produced more slowly in an old than in a young cell or even may be broken down more rapidly in the aging cell.

And investigators at the Gerontology Research Center and elsewhere are trying to see whether the number of receptors in old cells can be restored to the level of young cells, overcoming some of the effects of hormone deficiencies that come with aging.

Receptors are now being purified, and studies on their production and degradation are under way. And there is beginning to be evidence that increasing the number of receptors in old cells is possible.

For example, at the Ethel Percy Andrus Gerontology Center at the University of Southern California, a brilliant young neurobiologist, Dr. Caleb Finch, in studies after giving female mice estrogen injections, found that the injections increased the number of estrogen receptors in the mice's uteri.

Says Dr. Roth: "With the exciting knowledge that certain hormones can regulate their own as well as other receptors, the possibility for manipulation of responsiveness during aging must now be taken seriously."

Meanwhile, Dr. Finch also is working on another potentially important aspect of the aging phenomenon. He believes that the brain has important "pacemaker functions" for controlling the rate of aging of body systems.

Finch and others have noted that certain areas of the brain, such as the hypothalamus, actually control the activities of the master gland at the base of the brain, the pituitary, in sending hormonal instructions to various systems of the body.

Almost all bodily systems depend upon stimulation by pituitary hormones. The pituitary earned its designation as the body's master gland because it was long believed to be independent. But more recently the pituitary has been found to depend for its proper functioning on signals it receives from the hypothalamus.

In his work with animals, Dr. Finch has found that as an animal ages there are changes in the transmission mechanisms within the hypothalamus which can influence the brain area's control over the pituitary.

It is possible, Finch and others believe, to work on improving the situation either by improving the precision with which the hypothalamus signals the pituitary or by remedying the failure of the pituitary by supplying from outside what the pituitary is failing to produce.

The Immune System

Meanwhile, at the Baltimore Center and elsewhere, many scientists have been studying what happens to the body's immune system with aging, what the consequences are, and what might be done to overcome them.

Ordinarily, the immune system produces antibodies that have the job of recognizing and attacking invading viruses, bacteria, and other foreign agents. Additionally, evidence is growing that they are responsible for detecting and destroying incipient cancer cells as they arise in the body.

For many years, investigators have known that the body's immune-system response decreases with age and that this is probably a major factor in the increased susceptibility of older people to infectious diseases and perhaps to malignancy.

Moreover, Sir Macfarlane Burnet of the University of Melbourne, one of the world's most distinguished scientists, as well as other investigators have shown that the body can also produce antibodies that instead of attacking invaders attack natural body tissues. Such autoantibodies, as they are called, are believed to be one cause of senility as well as of certain diseases, including rheumatoid arthritis, which have been labeled autoimmune diseases.

And it appears that with aging the immune system undergoes changes which lead to an increase in the level of autoantibodies even as the production of disease-fighting antibodies declines.

Several years ago, working at the National Institutes of Health in Bethesda, Maryland, Dr. Takashi Makinodan and his associates were able to measure how drastically immune-system efficiency can decline with age.

When they exposed laboratory animals to controlled doses of disease organisms in order to trigger immune-system defense, they found that the response in old animals was only 10 percent of the response in the young; the old animals had only one-tenth the capacity of the young to fight off infection. In man that could mean that a seventy-year-old may be ten times as open to disease as a teen-ager.

The problem may lie with the two types of cells that produce antibodies. These are T cells formed in the thymus gland and B cells formed in the bone marrow. When a foreign agent enters the body, one T cell and as many as eight B cells, join to form an immunocompetent unit, and it is this combined unit that produces antibodies. Makinodan and his group found that in old age the T and B cells do not diminish in numbers but are not as efficient in recognizing invaders, and they form as few as 20 percent of the normal number of immunocompetent units, each of which turns out only half as many antibodies as in youth.

In 1975, work at the Baltimore Center indicated that there may also be another contributing factor in the reduction of immunity with age—an increased number of cells that inhibit the protective activities of the body's immune response.

Promisingly, however, immunologists are searching for ways to enhance the activity of the immune system in people of all ages.

For example, at the University of California, Los Angeles, Dr. Roy Walford has placed laboratory animals on diets moderately restricted in calories or proteins which have not only increased resistance to some viral infections but also prolonged the animals' life spans and improved their resistance to certain tumors. Evidently, the immune systems of the animals on special diets stayed "younger" longer than the systems of the other animals.

And promisingly too, Dr. Makinodan and his group have found that when old and young T and B cells are mixed together, the old cells become able to make antibodies at the same rate as the young cells. The investigators infected young animals with disease bacteria to stimulate their immune systems, then extracted some of their T and B cells, froze them for several months, and, after thawing, injected them into old mice. Long after getting the injections, the old mice were infected with disease organisms lethal to other old mice—and they resisted infection.

Conceivably, humans could deposit T and B cells in frozen storage during youth and use them in old age to revitalize their immune systems. First, however, researchers must determine if they can successfully freeze and restore live human cells.

Another possible means of maintaining or restoring immune-system efficiency may come from the recent findings of Dr. Allan Goldstein and other researchers at the University of Texas Medical Branch, Galveston. The thymus gland, which lies behind the upper part of the breastbone extending into the neck, secretes a hormone, thymosin, only recently purified. The Texas workers have found that thymosin production declines with age and may contribute to aging by retarding the ability of the immune system to function effectively.

Having established that injections of thymosin in mice increase their immunity, Dr. Goldstein and his co-workers are hopeful they can establish that such injections may do the same in humans.

Free Radicals

The possibility that substances known as free radicals may influence aging is under study.

Free radicals are fragments of molecules that, in effect, have come unstuck. Eager to recombine, to find new molecular homes, they may react with anything nearby. Such free radical recombinations, called oxidative reactions, are behind many natural decay processes—such as the rancidification of butter and even some industrial processes such as the drying of oil paint. To counter free radical reactions and help preserve foods, antioxidant materials are used, which include vitamin E and BHT, a material often employed as a breakfast food preserver.

Free radicals are present in the human body, and some investigators believe they may play a role in aging within body cells. Dr. Denham Harman of the University of Nebraska School of Medicine has found that free radicals have a role in forming amyloid, a fibrous protein that can be seen in increasing amounts with age in blood vessels in the brain and in areas of cell degeneration in brain tissue. Conceivably, free radicals could be a factor in producing senility by damaging brain cells and vessels; and, by damaging other body cells and tissues, they could play a part in declining immune response and general aging.

In laboratory studies, Dr. Harman has fed mice on vitamin E and BHT and in some strains has achieved an increased average life span of as much as 50 percent.

Recently, too, Dr. Harman, studying immune responses, has

added to the diet of mice from age six weeks through eighty-eight weeks either vitamin E or a chemical, ethyoxyquin, which also inhibits free radical reactions. Both the additives were found to enhance immune responses. Subsequently, other free radical inhibitors—including levamisole, 2-mercaptoethyanol, butylated hydroxytoluene, 2-mercaptoethylamine, and sodium hypophosphite—proved effective.

These studies, as Dr. Harman and his colleagues have reported, suggest but do not prove that some free radical reactions contribute to the decline of the immune response with age and the decline can be ameliorated by adding inhibitors to the diet.

In still other work related to free radicals, Dr. Harman and his colleagues have been looking into the effect of dietary fat on nervous system functioning. Fat, a major component of most human diets, can participate in free radical reactions. In studies with animals, fat—some forms in particular—impeded the ability of rats to learn to go through a maze. The more unsaturated the fat, the greater the number of errors in maze-running. On the other hand, rats that were also given vitamin E in their diets performed significantly better.

Thus, suggest the investigators, variation in the amount or degree of unsaturated dietary fat consumed and of factors such as vitamin E that can modify free radical reactions with the fat may contribute to the variability between people in central nervous system changes such as senility.

Cross-Linking

Like leather and rubber, human skin and blood vessel walls tend to lose elasticity with age. The loss appears to be the result of a cross-linking process. Original elasticity comes from long fibers of a material called collagen. With time, chemical cross-links or hookups may be formed between the fibers, reducing their elasticity.

One avenue being explored by some researchers is a study

of how possibly a gradual chemical cross-linking in all body cells may contribute to aging.

Actually, cross-linkages are always being formed, and most of the time no harm is done, as body enzymes break up the linkages as fast as they are formed. But a certain percentage of cross-linkages may be formed in ways that prevent enzymes from splitting them, and as more and more are formed with time, normal cell functioning may deteriorate.

If this is true, can anything be done to minimize the formation of stubborn cross-linkages and to split up those already formed? A leader in cross-linkage research, Dr. Johan Bjorksten of the Bjorksten Research Foundation, Madison, Wisconsin, believes that both prophylaxis and therapy are possible.

For one thing, Bjorksten reports, oxidation of unsaturated fats in the body can lead to the formation of certain compounds, such as aldehydes, ketones, peroxides, and epoxides that are known to be potent cross-linking agents. These may be minimized either by controlling the intake of unsaturated fats or by use of an antioxidant such as vitamin E. What has to be determined is how much antioxidant can be used so that there is a protective effect without slowing down normal oxidation reactions to the point of making metabolism sluggish.

Dietary excesses, too, may be involved in cross-linkage, Bjorksten points out. If the amount of any nutrient ingested at any time exceeds the quantity which can be immediately processed at any step of metabolism, the intermediate product derived from that nutrient to that point accumulates and may spill into the bloodstream or to other sites where it should not be, causing undesirable reactions, the most damaging of which may be cross-linking.

"Cross-linking caused by metabolic intermediates," says Dr. Bjorksten, "could well be a principal reason why being overweight affects longevity so unfavorably. It is more judicious to take nutrition in many smaller meals than in a few large ones. This should help avoid overloading any metabolic step at any time and should reduce the amount of cross-linking agents formed."

Can cross-linkage be reversed? Some investigators, including Bjorksten, believe that this could become feasible. What is needed is to find enzymes capable of breaking down cross-linkages that cannot be split apart by natural body enzymes.

One source for such enzymes could be soil bacteria. It seems to some investigators that soil bacteria must contain suitable enzymes for the purpose, or the earth otherwise would remain covered with the undecomposed bodies of animals.

And, indeed, some microbes producing enzymes having such effects have been found. One of these bacterial enzymes, from a strain of Bacillus cereus, has been purified to a high degree. In test-tube studies, it has shown ability to dissolve the major portion of otherwise insoluble matter isolated from human brains and kidneys. It remains to be seen whether it can be used safely and effectively in the human body.

All of the research work discussed here represents only a small part of the total investigational effort now in progress. And the total can be expected to grow—vastly and rapidly—now that aging has begun to be almost a "glamour" area of biomedical research and research funds are increasing.

A Selected Bibliography

1. Senility: Fear, Fancy, Fact

Savitz, H. A. Mental Hygiene for the Aged. *New York State Journal of Medicine* 76:1850.

Butler, R. N. Successful Aging. *MH (Mental Hygiene)* 58 (3):6.

2. The Changes That Do—and Do Not—Occur with Aging

Human Aging II. Department of Health, Education, and Welfare Publication No. (HSM) 71–9037:61.

Birren J. E., in *Aging: Prospects and Issues.* University of Southern California Press, 1973.

Haydu, G. G. Aging and Experience Forms. *New York State Journal of Medicine* 75:1556.

Sherman, E. David. Retirement. *Journal of the American Geriatrics Society* 18:780.

Wallace, D. J. The Biology of Aging. *Journal of the American Geriatrics Society* 25:104.

Busse, E. W. Physiological Changes and Disease, in Exton-Smith, A. N., and Evans, J. G., editors. *Care of the Elderly.* London: Academic Press, 1977.

The Normality of Aging: The Baltimore Longitudinal Study. National Institute on Aging Science Writer Seminar Series.

Lamy, P. P., and Kitler, M. E. The Geriatric Patient: Age-Dependent Physiologic and Pathologic Changes. *Journal of the American Geriatric Society* 19:871.

Diamond, M. C. The Aging Brain: Some Enlightening and Optimistic Results. *American Scientist* 66:66.

3. True Senility (Dementia)

Editorial: Dementia. *Medical Tribune* 19 (9):11.

Samorajski, T. How the Human Brain Responds to Aging. *Journal of the American Geriatrics Society* 24:4.

Alzheimer's Disease Conference. *NIH Record,* July 12, 1977, p. 4.

Liston, E. H., Jr. Occult Presenile Dementia. *Journal of Nervous and Mental Disease* 164:263.

Manuelidis, E. E., et al. Viremia in Experimental Creutzfeldt-Jakob Disease. *Science* 200:1069.

"Rare" Alzheimer's "Identical" to Usual Senile Dementia. *Medical Tribune* 18 (26):3.

Rx of Concurrent Disease Eases Dementia. *Medical Tribune* 19 (4):3.

4. The Pseudosenilities (Pseudodementias)

Hyperlipidemic Dementia. Report to American Academy of Neurology by Dr. N. T. Mathew, Baylor College of Medicine, Houston.

Duckworth, G. S., and Ross, H. Diagnostic Differences in Psychogeriatric Patients in Toronto, New York, and London, England. *Canadian Medical Association Journal* 112:847.

Wells, C. E. Chronic Brain Disease: An Overview. *American Journal of Psychiatry* 135:1.

Charlton, M. H. Presenile Dementia. *New York State Journal of Medicine* 74:1493.

Reichel, W. Multiple Problems in the Elderly. *Hospital Practice* 3/76:103.

Adams, R. D., et al. Symptomatic Occult Hydrocephalus with "Normal" Cerebrospinal Fluid Pressure. *New England Journal of Medicine* 273:117.

Rice, E., and Gendelman, S. Psychiatric Aspects of Normal Pressure Hydrocephalus. *Journal of the American Medical Association* 223:409.

Rosen, H., and Swigar, M. E. Depression and Normal Pressure Hydrocephalus. *Journal of Nervous and Mental Disease* 163:35.

The "Senile" without Brain Atrophy May Be Treatable. "Medical News," *Journal of the American Medical Association* 232 (1):11.

Angel, R. W. Understanding and Diagnosing Senile Dementia. *Geriatrics* 8/77:47.

5. When It's a Matter of Brain Circulation

Cerebrovascular Dementia Reversible by Anastomosis. *Medical Tribune* 17 (18):43.

Dementia and Atherosclerosis. "Overseas Report," *Canadian Medical Association Journal* 111:1058.

Surgery Helps Mental Status of Some Patients. "Medical News," *Journal of the American Medical Association* 236:2037.

Leonberg, S. C., Jr., and Elliott, F. A. Preventing Stroke After TIA. *American Family Physician* 17 (1):179.

Ausman, J. E., et al. Brain Artery By-Pass Reduces Stroke Damage, Risk of Recurrence. Report from American Heart Association.

Fein, Jack M. Microvascular Surgery for Stroke. *Scientific American* 4/78:59.

Walsh, P. N., et al. Platelet Coagulant Activities and Serum Lipids in Transient Cerebral Ischemia. *New England Journal of Medicine* 295:854.

Steele, P., et al. Effect of Sulfinpyrazone on Platelet Survival Time in Patients with Transient Cerebral Ischemic Attacks. *Stroke* 8:396.

Editorial: Of Platelets, Their Antagonists, and Transient Cerebral Ischemia. *Journal of the American Medical Association* 239:228.

Rao, D. B., and Norris, J. R. A Double-Blind Investigation of Hydergine in the Treatment of Cerebrovascular Insufficiency in the Elderly. *Johns Hopkins Medical Journal* 130:317.

Rao, D. B., et al. Cyclandelate in the Treatment of Senile Mental Changes: A Double-Blind Evaluation. *Journal of the American Geriatrics Society* 25:548.

Gaitz, C. M., et al. Pharmacotherapy for Organic Brain Syndrome in Late Life. *Archives of General Psychiatry* 34:839.

Walsh, A. C., and Walsh, B. H. Presenile Dementia: Further Experience with an Anticoagulant-Psychotherapy Regimen. *Journal of the American Geriatrics Society* 22:467.

Psychochemical Treatment Counteracts Senility. *Science News* 111:292.

6. The Heart, the Blood, and the Mind

Congestive Heart Failure, in Likoff, W., et al. *Your Heart: Complete Information for the Family.* Philadelphia: Lippincott, 1972.

Abnormal Heart Rhythms. idem.

Anemia, in Galton, L. *The Disguised Disease: Anemia.* New York: Crown, 1975.

Giant Cell Arteritis May Be Relatively Common. "Medical News," *Journal of the American Medical Association* 217:1036.

Lewis, K. B. Heart Disease in the Elderly. *Hospital Practice* 2/76:99.

McCabe, E. S. Polymyalgia Rheumatica. *Journal of the American Geriatric Society* 24:89.

7. Turning Down the Pressure

Wilkie, F., and Eisdorfer, C. Intelligence and Blood Pressure in the Aged. *Science* 172:959.

Galton, L. *The Silent Disease: Hypertension.* New York: Crown, 1973.

Gifford, R. W. There Is a Case for Treating Hypertension in the Elderly. Symposium on Recent Advances in Management and Prevention of Cardiovascular Disease, sponsored by Bowman Gray School of Medicine.

Mahler, H. Down with High Blood Pressure. *World Health* 2–3/ 78:2.

8. Solving the Gland Problems

Whybrow, P. C., et al. Mental Changes Accompanying Thyroid Gland Dysfunction. *Archives of General Psychiatry* 20:48.

Tsao, J. M., and Catz, B. Disguised Thyroid Disorders. *California Medicine* 103:91.

Cremer, G. M., et al. University of North Carolina Thyroid Studies. *Neurology* 19:37.

Barnes, B. O., and Galton, L. *Hypothyroidism: The Unsuspected Illness.* New York: Crowell, 1976.

Davis, P. J. Endocrines and Aging. *Hospital Practice* 9/77:113.

9. Detecting and Eliminating the Depressive Influence

Gianturco, D. T., and Busse, E. W. Psychiatric Problems Encountered During a Long-Term Study of Normal Ageing Volunteers, in Isaacs, A. D., and Post, F., editors. *Studies in Geriatric Medicine.* London: John Wiley & Sons.

Joffe, J. R. Functional Disorders in the Elderly. *Hospital Practice* 6/76:93.

Cammer, L. What's New and Important About Depression. "In Consultation," *Medical Tribune* 17 (35):7.

Fieve, R. R. What's New and Important About Lithium. "In Consultation," *Medical Tribune* 18 (2):16.

Learning About Depressive Illnesses. National Institute of Mental Health, DHEW Publication No. (HSM) 72–9110.

Bowers, M. B. Clinical Aspects of Depression in a Home for the Aged. *Journal of the American Geriatrics Society* 17:469.

Cole, M. G., and Muller, H. F. Sleep Deprivation in the Treatment of Elderly Depressed Patients. *Journal of the American Geriatrics Society* 24:308.

10. Halting the Drug-Induced Pseudosenilities

Gilbert, G. J. Quinidine Dementia. *Journal of the American Medical Association* 237:2093.

Krebs, H. On the Overuse and Misuse of Medication. *Executive Health* 11 (2).

Lamy, P. P., and Kitler, M. E. Drugs and the Geriatric Patient. *Journal of the American Geriatric Society* 19:23.

Korcok, M. Drugs and the Elderly: University of Miami Symposium. *Canadian Medical Association Journal* 118:1320.

Reichel, W. Organic Brain Syndromes in the Aged. *Hospital Practice* 5/76:119.

Achong, M. R., et al. Prescribing of Psychoactive Drugs for Chronically Ill Elderly Patients. *Canadian Medical Association Journal* 118:1503.

Ruedy, J. Monitoring Drug Use. *Canadian Medical Association Journal* 118:1483.

Hall, R. C. W., and Kirkpatric, B. The Benzodiazepines. *American Family Physician* 17 (5):131.

Galton, L. Symptoms from Drugs, in *The Complete Book of Symptoms and What They Mean.* New York: Simon & Schuster, 1978.

11. Overcoming the Deficiency-Triggered

Mitra, M. L. Confusional States in Relation to Vitamin Deficiencies in the Elderly. *Journal of the American Geriatrics Society* 19:536.

Malnutrition a Problem in U.S. Hospitals. *Modern Medicine* 46 (8):16.

Rao, D. B. Problems of Nutrition in the Aged. *Journal of the American Geriatrics Society* 21:362.

Schuster, M. M. Disorders of the Aging GI System. *Hospital Practice* 9/76:95.

McCann, M. B., and Foell, K. M. Nutrition for the Elderly. *The New Physician* 6/78:41.

Butler, R. N. Nutrition and Aging. Statement before the Select Committee on Nutrition and Human Needs of the U.S. Senate, September 23, 1977.

The Unexplored Frontiers of Nutrition in the 1980's. Remarks by Dr. M. Rupert Cutler, Assistant Secretary of Agriculture, at National Institute of Health Conference, "The Research Basis of Clinical Nutrition," Bethesda, Maryland, June 20, 1978.

12. And Still Other Correctables

Klawans, H. L., and Topel, J. L. "Falling Disease." Report from Michael Reese Medical Center, Chicago.

Wells, C. E. Transient Ictal Psychosis. *Archives of General Psychiatry* 32:1201.

Ruben, R. J. Otolaryngologic Problems of the Old. *Hospital Practice* 8/77:73.

Hoogerbeets, J. D., and LaWall, J. Changing Concepts of Psychiatric Problems in the Aged. *Geriatrics* 8/75:83.

Eckstein, D. Common Complaints of the Elderly. *Hospital Practice* 4/76:67.

Hunt, T. E. Rehabilitation of the Elderly. *Hospital Practice* 1/ 77:89.

Sachs, A. E. Major General Surgery in the Geriatric Population. *Journal of Abdominal Surgery* 11/74:314.

13. The Matter of Vigor

Randolph, J. You Are Never Too Old to Feel Young. Congressional Record, Vol. 116, No. 210.

DeCarlo, T. J., et al. A Program of Balanced Physical Fitness in the Preventive Care of Elderly Ambulatory Patients. *Journal of the American Geriatrics Society* 25:331.

Ochsner, A. Aging. *Journal of the American Geriatrics Society* 24:385.

Exercise and Aging. Physical Fitness Research Digest of the President's Council on Physical Fitness and Sports, Series 7, No. 2.

De Vries, H. A., et al. National Institute on Aging Symposium on Exercise and Aging. *Medical Tribune* 19 (1):1, 19 (2):19.

14. The Right Help When It's Needed

Charatan, F. B. Somebody DO Something . . . about the Mistreatment of Elderly Patients. *Modern Medicine* 3/15/78:35.

Outcalt, D. Treating the Elderly. "The President's Column," *The New Physician* 26 (11):71.

Goldstein, S. The Music of Time: A Plea for More Gerontology Resources. *Canadian Medical Association Journal* 118:966.

Harman, D. The Clinical Gerontologist. *Journal of the American Geriatrics Society* 24:452.

Hyams, D. E. Teaching Geriatric Medicine. *New York State Journal of Medicine* 77:2241.

Rao, D. B. The Team Approach to Integrated Care of the Elderly. *Geriatrics* 32:88.

Butler, R. N. Medicine and Aging. Testimony before the Senate Special Committee on Aging, October 13, 1976.

Pennington, F. C., et al. Continuing Medical Education in Geriatrics. *New York State Journal of Medicine* 77:2105.

15. The Frontiers

Marx, J. L. Learning and Behavior: Effects of Pituitary Hormones. *Science* 190:367.

Wurtman, R. J. Food for Thought. *The Sciences* (N.Y. Academy of Sciences) 18 (4):6.

Davis, K. L., et al. Physostigmine: Improvement of Long-Term Memory Processes in Normal Humans. *Science* 201:272.

Sitaram, N., and Weingartner, H. Human Serial Learning: Enhancement with Arecholine and Choline and Impairment with Scopolamine. *Science* 201:274.

Roth, G. S. Hormone Receptor Changes During Adulthood and Senescence: Significance for Aging Research. *Federation Proceedings* (in press).

Nordin, A. A., and Makinodan, T. Humoral Immunity in Aging. *Federation Proceedings* 33:2033.

Adler, W. H. Aging and Immune Function. *BioScience* 25:652.

Samorajski, T. Central Neurotransmitter Substances and Aging: A Review. *Journal of the American Geriatrics Society* 25:337.

Harman, D. H., et al. Free Radical Theory of Aging: Effect of Free-Radical-Reaction Inhibitors on the Immune Response. *Journal of the American Geriatrics Society* 25:400.

Bjorksten, J. The Crosslinkage Theory of Aging: Clinical Implications. *Comprehensive Therapy* 2 (2):65.

Butler, R. N. Research Programs of the National Institute on Aging. Public Health Reports, U.S. Department of Health, Education, and Welfare 92 (1):3.

Index